The following r ... ve followed Freda Whalen's program:

Thanks for the guidance and information I have received from you personally and also from your book. Having been on your program for about six weeks, I can truthfully say that I feel so much better.

—J. David, Lake Charles, LA

At first I was quite skeptical about trying Freda's program but nothing else worked so I followed her advice. Within a couple of months, to my surprise, I felt much better. The diet of complex carbohydrates backed up with protein as Freda suggested along with the vitamin supplements and an exercise program made a tremendous difference.

—T. Frame, Opelousas, LA

I got on Freda's program over 10 years ago. She has helped me to understand how to balance my foods and look for the hidden sugars, all of which have made a remarkable difference in my health. Please feel free to use this in your book Freda. I want others to know that they, too, can get results from your program.

—C. G. Mcdonald, Lake Charles, LA

I was diagnosed with hypoglycemia five years ago. Until I met Freda, I had thought I would never feel good again. When I first tried her suggestions I was amazed how good I felt. I could think better, had more energy and wasn't depressed all the time. After about three months on her program I didn't think I had hypoglycemia anymore so one day at a party I decided to eat everything! I didn't feel too bad after my big splurge and that was when I decided that my hypoglycemia was gone. After a few weeks off the program I began to realize how often I was craving sweets again, and my headaches started coming back. For a while I was ashamed to go back to Freda, To my surprise she was very understanding. Once again she helped me to work my way back to her program and once again I am feeling good. I learned my lesson, Freda does know the problems we face because she has been there. Thanks Freda for your love and support, I could not have done it without you. I hope someone else will have as much help from your program as I have.

—B. Gilley, Hornbeck, LA

I am very grateful to Freda. Her program did work and still does, as long as I stay with it. I have used her suggestions, recipes, and her first book over and over again. I will always be indebted to her for better health.

—J. Mayo, Lake Charles, LA

Hypoglycemia and Diabetes Wellness Guide

by

Freda Whalen, RMT
(registered massage therapist)

with Gilbert Manso, M.D.

Edited by Colin Ingram

Body Care Publications • Lake Charles, Louisiana

The difference in the dietary approach contained in this book is the balancing of complex carbohydrates with adequate levels of complete proteins in order to achieve and maintain a balance of blood sugars in hypoglycemia and diabetic conditions.

Make this book a way of life.
Use it, live by it,
but never loan it to a friend.
You will never get it back.

CONTENTS

ACKNOWLEDGEMENTS

I am especially indebted to Dr. Gilbert Manso, MD. for his generous contribution to this book. Without his support and medical expertise, this book would not have been possible. Many thanks to Dr. L. R. Savoie, OD, for his continued support in my work throughout these last five years, and for his unselfishness in giving of his valuable time for lectures to our support groups.

Thanks to my my family for their faith in me. Special thanks to my daughters, Carla, Vickie and Christina for their talents and energies and for helping me to complete and realize my dream. Also thanks to my sisters, Willie Dean Mansel and Rita Hurd, for all their ideas and support.

I would also like to take this opportunity to thank Colin Ingram for his work and dedication to my goal of producing a near-perfect product. Like a sculptor, he shaped the raw materials of four years of hard work into a masterpiece. Colin, you are truly a master of your art.

As always, I thank God for His help in enabling me to take charge of my own body and for giving me the strength to continue in my efforts to find a better, healthier way of life so that I may help others to do the same.

Proof Reader
£

THE AUTHORS

A hypoglycemic herself, **Freda Whalen** has helped many others further their understanding of how to cope with this confusing and often misunderstood disease.

She is a nationally accredited AFAA (Aerobics and Fitness Association of America) Aerobics and Fitness Instructor; she is a Certified Nutritionist through the National Institute of Nutritional Education, in Aurora, CO; Freda is also a Massage Therapist, nationally certified by the AMTA (American Massage Therapy Association) and licensed by the State of Texas and Louisiana.

She has a full and demanding private practice as a Personal Fitness Trainer and a Massage Therapist. She also teaches courses in nutrition and injury prevention, and has lead Hypoglycemia Support Groups in several major cities.

A native of Mamou, Louisiana, she now resides and practices in Lake Charles, Louisiana.

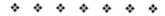

Dr. Gilbert Manso received his Bachelor's degree from the University of Texas in Austin and his Medical Doctorate from the University of Texas School of Medicine in Galveston. He is on the teaching faculty at the University of Texas Medical School in Houston, is Board Certified in Family Practice and is a Fellow of the American College of Family Practice.

Dr. Manso lived in Cuba for fifteen years; in addition, he practiced medicine one year in Asia and four years in Europe.

He practices holistic medicine, and has maintained a special interest in the treatment of hypoglycemia, candida yeast, digestive and chronic problems in adults and children. He has been in private practice in Houston, Texas since 1975.

Foreword

No one starts a journey without first having a destination or a road map. *Hypoglycemia and Diabetes Wellness Guide* offers you, the reader, a road map to a healthier life through better nutrition and a healthier lifestyle.

Millions of people suffer with blood sugar disorders that are often misdiagnosed, misunderstood, or seem unimportant to many health care professionals. Many people are trapped, with no where to turn, because so few professionals understand these illnesses or how to treat them.

By the year 2,000 there will be an estimated 268.1 million people with blood sugar disorders in the United States. Out of this number some 34 million will have diabetes and twice as many will have hypoglycemia. Approximately 100 million people may have some form of blood sugar disorder. Possibly, one person in three will need to seriously alter his or her dietary habits to maintain control of blood sugar levels, in order to enjoy a happier, healthier life.

More than ever, people are realizing the need for healthier approaches in preventing disease through better nutrition. Most of us are searching for better ways to cope with our health problems.

While the diabetic may use medications such as insulin to help control his or her blood sugar levels, unfortunately, the hypoclycemic does not have this option. Only a controlled diet and a healthier lifestyle will help him or her to balance and control blood sugar levels.

Having lived with hypoglycemia for fifteen years, Freda Whalen has a unique understanding of the many problems people face each day as hypoglycemics. Through strong will and determination, she has been able to take control of her life and her destiny. She has been able to operate a successful neuromuscular therapeutic massage clinic, a health food store, and (at the age of fifty) she has found the time and energy to complete her third book, *Hypoglycemia and Diabetes Wellness Guide.*

With complete physician endorsement, this book explores various aspects of diet, exercise, and ways to control the many challenges associated with hypoglycemia and diabetes. The authors have combined personal experience with medical research to help clarify and identify the symptoms of these blood sugar disorders. They discuss causes of the disorders and they offer ways to live with hypoglycemia and diabetes and still feel great.

You will learn that on rare occasions when hypoglycemia is correctly diagnosed, the medical advice given may actually be the opposite of what is needed to control this disease. To temporarily alleviate symptoms, doctors frequently prescribe treatment which may perpetuate the disease.

This book provides a plan to successfully control blood sugar disorders. It offers a guide for better nutrition, an exercise plan for total fitness, and effective ways to improve your lifestyle and mental attitude.

At times, most of us are tempted to eat foods that contain refined sugar—even though we may know that we cannot tolerate them. Many people are completely unaware of "hidden" sugars in foods. This book provides the hypoglycemic and diabetic with alternatives to eating unhealthy foods which contain refined sugars and refined carbohydrates. All of the recipes in this book are created with complex carbohydrates, which are similar to the foods that we have enjoyed throughout our lives.

The majority of people who have hypoglycemia do not know it and they may have given up on living a normal, happy life. Now based on her extensive work with hypoglycemia, Freda Whalen and co-author, Gilbert Manso, M.D., have written a practical, "how to" guide that describes ways to set up an individual, therapeutic program and suggests ways to maintain this healthy program for life.

INTRODUCTION

Like most of you, when I was younger I believed life was forever, and weakness and illness were something that happened to other people, not to me. Nutrition never entered my thoughts and it never occurred to me that sugar was not healthy. Not having a weight problem, counting calories was of no concern and there wasn't the concern over low cholesterol and low fat diets that we are now aware of today.

As a child, I remember having severe migraine headaches and an inability to cope with stress. In the years that followed, migraine headaches, low energy, nervousness and insomnia became more and more of a problem for me. The midnight cravings for sugar became uncontrollable, especially around my ovulation time. I had so many sleepless nights I thought of myself as a night person. Much of my housework and household chores were accomplished between the hours of midnight and four in the morning. Exhausted, I would drift off into a fitful sleep only to be awakened all too soon by that faithful alarm clock. Needless to say, I wasn't at by best in those days. The combination of stress and improper nutrition was taking its toll on my health.

I was diagnosed with hypoglycemia in 1975. A co-worker had mentioned hypoglycemia as a possible explanation for all the problems I was having, so on my insistence my physician ordered a glucose tolerance test. Even though the test turned out positive, my doctor informed me that I should not concern myself with the diagnosis. Many people went through life without any apparent problems with this condition. I was told to have something containing sugar with me at all times. If I felt weak or nervous, the sugar would bring my blood level to normal and I

1

should do fine. Of course, I took my physician's advise. But it wasn't long before I noticed how often I felt weak or nervous. The sugar helped me for a while but no one had mentioned anything about the awful let-down feeling I was beginning to feel with each passing day. The more sugar I ate, the more I craved and the symptoms of hypoglycemia continued to get worse. The anxiety and panic attacks that had long been a problem also increased. I had no understanding as to why I would react in certain situations in such panic. Many days all I wanted to do was sit in a dark room curled up in a chair, not wanting to talk to anyone.

To add to my problems, the chronic urethritis with which I had suffered over the past thirteen years continued to build up. I could go no longer than a week or so without having a urethra dilation. In the course of two years it was necessary to have two surgeries on my bladder to remove scar tissue caused from all the dilations. I was so dependent on Librax, valium and over-the-counter sleeping drugs that I could not face a day or night without them. It all became a vicious cycle.

We all have weaknesses. Mine had always been coconut cake, and my favorite midnight snack was Pepperidge Farms Coconut Layer Cake. Looking back now it is no wonder I was so ill. I am embarrassed to admit it, but I often ate the whole cake in those early morning hours. My afternoon snack of a box of chocolate covered cherries, a can of Pringles Potato Chips with a large coke became a ritual. I still did not associate all the cravings for sugar and the other health problems I was having with hypoglycemia.

Morning headaches were a way of life, especially on weekends when I slept late. There were times I was so fatigued I could hardly put one foot in front of the other. I knew something was very wrong with me, but I didn't know what it was. When I mentioned these problems to my doctor, I was told I was under too much stress and I should take my valium and learn to manage the stress in my life.

My mental confusion was such a problem that there were days I could not function. My mood swings were to the point that it was a wonder I had any friends left. I couldn't remember how to do the simple tasks I had done so often without thinking, like cooking or putting up my groceries in the pantry. I was afraid of getting out of the house. I couldn't recall how to get somewhere I had driven to many times before. I would get lost and at times could not remember my way back home.

I don't know how long I would have continued in this manner had I not been involved in a near accident. While running errands, I remember feeling weak and dizzy while driving. Luckily I stopped the car before blacking out. The next thing I realized someone was asking me if I was all right. The young man wanted to know if he could call anyone to help me or if he could do anything for me. I was so confused I did not even know my own name. I was so far out of it I know he must have thought I had been drinking. I can't remember how I finally made it home that day, but I knew something was very wrong with me and I had to get some help and some answers.

It was time for a yearly check-up, so I decided to find a new doctor. It had been two years since I had been diagnosed with hypoglycemia and I was beginning to believe that my blood sugar had something to do with the problems I had been having. In talking to my new doctor I was once again assured that I was doing the "right thing," eating sugar when I felt weak or nervous, and that the mental confusion I was experiencing did not have anything to do with the hypoglycemia. Before leaving his office he suggested I speak with a dietician at one of the hospitals for advice concerning my diet.

I left my appointment with the dietician feeling more confused and overwhelmed about my eating habits. I decided it was time I found out whatever I could about hypoglycemia. I had fooled around for the past two years in a complete fog; it was time I found out if there was anything I could do to help myself or at least understand what I was up against.

I stopped off at the public library. From that day on I have gone through an educational process I never dreamed could happen. I realized it was time I took responsibility for my own health. There was so much to learn, I was determined that this was not going to get the best of me.

After several weeks on a new diet, I was feeling better, but I knew I still had a long way to go. In order to have a better understanding of the foods I was eating, I kept a diary of all the foods I ate and the time schedule between meals. Whenever I had a headache, or my energy level was low, I could go back and check what I had actually eaten and how long it had been since my last meal. In every case there was an explanation for the problems I was having. Either I had eaten the wrong kinds of foods or I had gone too long between meals. I would then eliminate the food I had eaten with sugar, or make a note not to go as long between meals.

As my knowledge of foods improved, so did my health. My good days were more frequent, with fewer headaches and increased energy, and my determination to improve my health became the most important focus in my life. For too many years I had accepted my failing health as just the way it was supposed to be; no longer could I sit back and let others control my life.

Three months into my program I could see I had made the correct choice for myself. My family was amazed with the changes in my personality. This was a side they had never seen in me. I had more energy, more confidence in myself and felt alive for the first time in many years. Within six months, I knew I was on my way to a healthier life than I had ever thought possible. Even the chronic urethritis was no longer a problem. After all these years of undergoing those painful dilations it was a miracle not to have to go through that anymore. Everyone in my life could not help but notice the changes in my health.

The longer I was on my program, the more I understood that not only was sugar intake crucial, but overall proper nutrition was equally important. Not only did I want to be free from hypoglycemia symptoms, I wanted to be as healthy as I possibly could be. This meant changing even more of my bad habits.

Without realizing what was happening, other people with blood sugar problems started talking to me, asking questions about what I was doing to solve my problems with hypoglycemia.

Checking with the health unit in my area, I knew there were many support groups for other health problems, but none for hypoglycemia. So I decided, why not form our own group? I placed an announcement in the local newspaper and to my surprise over fifty hypoglycemics responded. I was amazed at the need for such a support group. Sharing ideas and recipes, and in general giving each other moral support, was a wonderfully rewarding experience. Plus, sharing my experience with others helped me to stay with my own program.

There were many times in these early years that I was tempted to give up my nutritional diet. One day I even went as far as buying a large cake, opening it up and just looking at it and smelling it for the longest time. But before taking my first bite, some good sense rushed to my rescue. I remembered how bad I used to feel and I just couldn't go through with it. It wasn't worth the price I would have to pay.

Since then I have spent many years helping people recognize and overcome their blood sugar problems. More and more I have realized that the average person is hungry for information on how to improve his/her health. Too often we have heard that our problem is only psychosomatic. We are prescribed anti-depressants, nerve pills, and even heart medications for the heart palpitations, instead of being helped with a good nutritional and fitness program.

I compare life to reading a book. Each page we turn is a new day in our lives and each time that page is turned, a new challenge is before us for that day. The pages turn into chapters and chapters into months until the book is completed. Each new book represents a year in our life. Whatever we have learned throughout that year gives us the knowledge and courage to face the challenges in our life.

The purpose of this book is to help you meet your challenges on a day-to-day basis.

I am not a physician, nor do I claim to be one. I am just an individual like yourself who got fed up feeling sick and tired, and decided to do something about it. Although I can't meet each of you in person, I want to reach you through this book. I want you to know that your symptoms, which may have been brushed aside by well-meaning medical practitioners, are real and valid; and that the knowledge to become well again is available. And lastly, I want each of you to have the energizing, satisfying, life-supporting experience of real wellbeing.

Freda Whalen

If I had known I would have lived this long,
I would have taken better care of myself.

—Anonymous

Do

Use this book to help alleviate sugar-related problems, which include hypoglycemia, diabetes, candida (yeast), hyperactive children, attention deficit disorder, fibromyalgia and obesity. This book will also be of benefit to those without sugar-related problems who want to begin an overall program of improving and maintaining their health.

Do share the information in this book with your doctor. Most traditional medical doctors are not familiar with these concepts of treating hypoglycemia and diabetes, and we encourage you to help them become familiar with this holistic approach.

Don't

Use this book in place of a doctor for diagnosing or treating any serious disease or specific condition. In particular, if there is a chance you may be suffering from diabetes, see your doctor.

Section I

General Information

CHAPTER 1

QUESTIONS AND ANSWERS

Whether in my private nutrition counseling or in my support group meetings, I am asked many questions by hypoglycemics and diabetics. Here are answers to some of the most frequently asked questions.

Q: *What role does stress play in diabetes and hypoglycemia?*
A: Stress causes the adrenal glands to react as in an emergency situation (the flight or fight syndrome). Stress also depletes vitamin B complex and vitamin C in the body, which are necessary for proper adrenal function. Both diabetics and hypoglycemics have a weak or depleted adrenal system, making it more difficult to cope with stressful situations. The adrenals also play a major role in the control of insulin released by the pancreas.

Q: *What role does exercise play in diabetes and hypoglycemia?*
A: There are two aspects to this. In general, exercise relieves stress, and the biochemistry of the body is improved through regular aerobic exercise. Exercise stimulates the endocrine system to function more efficiently and produce a normal hormonal output. This allows the

body to handle stress more effectively. Sleep patterns are also improved.

Exercise also causes changes in blood sugar and insulin levels. For hypoglycemics, exercise is very beneficial. For diabetics, exercise is also beneficial but it must be carefully coordinated with the timing and amount of insulin dosages. If you are a diabetic, be sure to have your doctor approve your exercise program before beginning it.

Q: *Why is fiber important in the diet?*
A: In addition to its other beneficial roles, fiber plays an important role in balancing blood sugar levels. Sugar and refined carbohydrates produce a high insulin release into the blood stream. which lowers the blood sugar too rapidly, causing a variety of symptoms. Fiber slows the conversion of foods into glucose, slowing and regulating the digestive process, maintaining a slower, steadier release of sugar into the blood stream.

Q: *How often should we have meals?*
A: When large amounts of foods are eaten at infrequent levels, the body responds to this excess of foods by releasing sudden bursts of insulin in order to counteract what the body sees as an imbalance in the system. This makes it impossible for the blood sugar to remain stabilized. To regulate blood sugar it is important to consume food energy as needed. By eating small, frequent meals you are giving your body a steady supply of energy without causing an abnormal response.

Q: *Is a sugar-free diet the best way to control hypoglycemia?*
A: The best diet for controlling hypoglycemia includes control of protein, complex carbohydrates, fats and fiber. This book includes thorough instructions for adopting a nutritionally-balanced diet.

Q: *Will it hurt me to have occasional lapses in my diet?*
A: Yes it will. You are striving to establish a delicate balance in your body. When you have occasional lapses by eating sugar, you are disrupting its balance and creating a destabilized metabolism whose effects can last for a long time.

Q: *Are the do-it-yourself glucose tolerance kits that are sold in drug stores any good, and do you recommend that people with suspected blood sugar symptoms use them?*
A: These kits do help diabetics to monitor glucose levels, but they are not helpful for hypoglycemics. In hypoglycemia, it isn't the level of

blood sugar that is significant, but how quickly that level drops. Therefore, these kits can be misleading for the hypoglycemic.

Q: *If I currently have no symptoms, how important is it for me to begin a program of nutrition and fitness?*

A: An effective nutritional and fitness program will have an across-the-board benefit for all aspects of your health—now and in the future. The sooner you begin, the greater your chance of warding off disease and disabling conditions

Q: *Are diabetes and hypoglycemia inherited disorders?*

A: In many cases, yes. Family histories play a major role in whether or not you will have either of these disorders. On the other hand, scientists have shown that laboratory rats, when fed diets high in sugar and fats develop diabetes and other disorders regardless of inherited tendencies.

Q: *What are "hidden sugars" and how do I know when I am getting these in my diet?*

A: Hidden sugars are sugars that are called by other names, such as dextrose, sucrose and corn sweeteners. Because a product does not list "sugar" in its ingredients does not mean it is sugar-free. This book provides the information you need to avoid hidden sugars.

Q: *Are diabetes and hypoglycemia ever cured?*

A: Work on identifying the genes that cause diabetes and hypoglycemia is accelerating, but at present there is no complete cure. The symptoms can be controlled by maintaining the proper diet and lifestyle, and it is the purpose of this book to help you do this so you can have a healthy and productive life.

CHAPTER 2

DESCRIPTION AND SYMPTOMS

Hypoglycemia

We recognize Diabetes as a disease, and it is time we recognize Hypoglycemia as a disease as well. Hypoglycemia is a condition of our "civilization" and is basically unknown in more primitive countries. Hypo means low and glycemia means sugar: low blood sugar. Diabetes is the opposite; it is high blood sugar, or hyper glycemia. Although diametrically opposed, they are closely related. Both are caused by the body's inability to metabolize sugar effectively.

Many of our physicians believe that hypoglycemia is relatively rare and most often occurs only in diabetics who use insulin or other blood sugar-lowering medications. Occasionally they will admit that hypoglycemia sometimes occurs in non-diabetics, but are quick to say that it rarely happens. Since there are several kinds of hypoglycemia, it is hard to find any two physicians who will agree or admit that hypoglycemia is a serious problem in this country. Hypoglycemics are often thought by physicians to be hypochondriacs or neurotics. And, in fact, hypoglycemia can mimic many other neuro-psychiatric disorders.

Therefore, it is hard to properly diagnose. Patients have been misdiagnosed as having such illnesses as schizophrenia, manic depressive psychosis, and psychopathic personalities. Many of the patients in our mental institutions and criminals in our society may be undiagnosed hypoglycemics. Studies have shown that many of these misunderstood, confused individuals are in desperate need of nutritional and medical attention.

The different kinds of hypoglycemia can be confusing. Fasting Hypoglycemia, which causes a low blood sugar level after 24 hours or longer of not eating, is rare and is caused by insulin-producing tumors in the pancreas. When our physicians tell us that hypoglycemia is a very rare disease, this is most likely the kind that they are referring to.

The absence of a counter-regulatory hormone called plasma glycogen is also a cause of hypoglycemia, and is another relatively rare form of this disease.

By far the most common form of hypoglycemia is Reactive Hypoglycemia, sometimes called Functional Hypoglycemia. This form is not only the most common, it is the one that is most often misdiagnosed.

Hypoglycemia can have such a wide range of symptoms, as shown in the following list, that it is easy to see why it is so often misdiagnosed. If you are a hypoglycemic, you may have many of the following symtoms or just a few.

Symptoms of Hypoglycemia

- Fits of anger
- Ringing in the ears
- Noise and light sensitivity
- Forgetfulness
- Trembling (shaking) of the hands
- Nervousness
- Magnify insignificant details
- Constant worrying
- Mental confusion
- Craving for sweets
- Obesity
- Dizziness, light-headed, fainting or blackouts
- Unconsciousness
- Difficulty in concentration
- Moodiness
- Allergies, asthma, skin rash, sinus trouble, etc.
- Itching and crawling sensation on skin

- Nightmares
- Chronic fatigue
- Fatigue relieved by eating
- Depressed (for no apparent reason)
- Headaches
- Insomnia or waking up after only a few hours sleep
- Sleepy during the day or after meals
- Can't get started in the mornings
- Phobias
- Anxiety attacks
- Suicidal thoughts; feeling of hopelessness
- Sighing or yawning
- Shortness of breath
- Hungry between meals or at night
- Shakiness or faint feeling before meals
- Can't decide things easily
- Low self-image
- Highly emotional
- Feel like you NEED an alcoholic drink
- Feel like you NEED that lift from coffee or Coke
- Eat when nervous
- Heart palpitations (heart beats fast)
- Bruise easily
- Reduced sex drive
- Unsocial behavior
- Eyes twitching
- Blurred vision
- Convulsions
- Hallucinations
- PMS (Pre-Menstrual Syndrome)

Symptoms of hypoglycemia are mainly due to the drop in blood sugar level after eating—they aren't caused by a steady, low blood sugar level. Therefore to determine absolutely whether or not you are hypoglycemic, you'll need to take a 5-6 hour glucose tolerance test.

The physician's interpretation of this test can make all the difference in the correct diagnosis and treatment. The standard medical procedure is to consider levels of blood sugar lower than 60 to 80 mg. per 100 ml. as hypoglycemia. Many physicians still believe that if your blood sugar doesn't drop lower than 50 mg., you don't have hypoglycemia. But physicians knowledgeable about hypoglycemia know that it is not how low the blood sugar drops, but how fast it drops that makes the difference.

If you should take a 5-6 hour glucose tolerance test, it is also important to chart your symptoms during the test. This way a complete evaluation of your condition can be made.

Your symptoms are an important indicator. One person may have severe symptoms from a given drop in sugar level, while another individual will be symptom-free with that same sugar level.

If you have an abnormally rapid drop in blood sugar after eating, and you are symptom-free, you may find that hypoglycemia symptoms occur at times of extra stress. If this should happen, you will have a pretty good idea of their cause.

Diabetes

If you are a diabetic, it is necessary that you are as careful as a hypoglycemic in avoiding all sugars. A diabetic cannot tolerate sugar any better than a hypoglycemic. When I counsel a diabetic client, I always recommend avoiding even fruits, fruit sweeteners and artificial sweeteners for several months, in order to help purify the system. It usually takes this long for the blood sugar to stabilize. We then slowly add a few raw fruits back into the diet. Concentrating on a high fiber diet and keeping the intake of the natural sugars down (as well as refined sugars) as much as possible is very important for all diabetics. As with hypoglycemia, it is important to eat at least six to eight small meals per day, keeping in mind that food is your fuel, and that your body needs a steady, but not overly large, supply.

Once your blood sugar has stabilized, you can usually add a sugar-free dessert every now and then, but never on a regular basis.

The diabetic patient has been given a false sense of security with the use of drugs like insulin. Insulin is often necessary, of course, in controlling blood sugar levels, but it isn't the answer to all of your problems. Degeneration at the cellular level is continuously taking place, making a total nutritional program even more important.

Since my area of knowledge is focused on hypoglycemia, I would like to introduce Dr. Gilbert Manso, to augment the information on diabetes.

Description, Symptoms and Control of Diabetes (Dr. Gilbert Manso)

There are several types of diabetes, but we are only going to discuss adult-onset diabetes mellitus. This is the most common form of diabetes, the one that appears after childhood. It is also called Type 2, and most recently, Non-Insulin Dependent Diabetes Mellitus (NIDDM). As the name implies, some Type 2 diabetics are not dependent on insulin.

There are several common early symptoms of diabetes. Some persons have only one of them while others have many of the following:

- Passing too much urine.
- Always thirsty.
- Increased hunger.
- Weight gain or weight loss, despite diet.
- Symptoms of hypoglycemia (see previous listing).
- Dizziness, particularly when getting up from lying or sitting.
- Mood changes.
- Fatigue.

A little later in the illness, one or more of the following symptoms usually appear:

- Changes in vision.
- Urine and bladder problems.
- Vaginal infections or itching.
- Indigestion, bloating or gas.
- Decreased sexual performance.
- Depression.
- Chronic fatigue.

Later on, vascular and nerve damage leads to muscle weakness and wasting, diarrhea, constipation, difficulty seeing, kidney failure, failure to heal, cataracts, blindness, strokes and heart attacks. Diabetes is the most common cause of blindness and kidney failure.

Type 2 Diabetes is frequently a nutritional illness and closely related to hypoglycemia. Early diabetes and hypoglycemia are both Impairments of Glucose Tolerance (IGT). In other words, the body's ability to tolerate or handle glucose (sugar) is impaired in diabetes and hypoglycemia.

The important environmental factors that lead to or aggravate IGT are:

1. Diet

2. Drugs

    - Alcohol and sugar
    - Cortisone (steroids)
    - Water pills (diuretics)

- Birth control pills
- Caffeine and nicotine
- Antibiotics

3. Stress

- Emotional
- Physical trauma
- Illness, fever

4. Digestive problems/liver problems

5. Physical inactivity

The diagnosis of diabetes is normally obvious from the patient's history and the physical examination. Laboratory tests confirm the diagnosis when the level of sugar in the blood is greater than 140 mg/dl on two different occasions. The person must not have had anything to eat for at least six (6) hours prior to this test, which is called "fasting blood sugar" or "FBS".

Sometimes the FBS test results are uncertain; then I do a "2-hour P. C. sugar," in which the blood is drawn two hours after a heavy lunch. If the 2-hour P. C. sugar is over 180, it strongly suggests diabetes.

Although rarely needed in testing for diabetes, another test, the 5-6 hour glucose tolerance test mentioned in the previous chapter, is sometimes needed to confirm this condition.

The treatment of diabetes requires more than diet, but diet is the cornerstone to the treatment. A treatment that does not include the diet and other elements presented in this book falls short of adequate.

In the following pages we have outlined many of the principles which I teach to most of my patients, not just diabetics. Many of the recipes I use are from the kitchen in my own office, where we cook daily for myself and the rest of my team. We incorporate these principles and diet into our own lives to help us stay healthy and productive.

The cornerstone of my treatment for most illnesses is to change the patient's lifestyle. This change must include a natural approach to nutrition and other aspects of living.

In diabetes and hypoglycemia, the diet is even more important than in most other illnesses. Although in some ways, hypoglycemia and diabetes are opposites in how the body reacts to sugar, in terms of diet their prevention and treatment are the same.

The basic principles of eating are:

1. Avoid artificial anything and additives. If God did not make it, do not eat it!

2. The less you do to a natural product before you eat it, the better. "Refined" products such as white flour and sugar are unhealthy.

3. Thou shall not eat fat. The less grease/oil/fat, the better.

4. The fewer animal products in the diet, the better. Do not eat meat products from pigs (ham, bacon, sausage). Fish that have fins and scales are the least harmful of the animal products.

5. If you are gaining weight, you are not eating right. You are either eating too much or you are eating the wrong foods or both.

6. Keep your diet simple.

After diet comes exercise. The benefits of regular exercise for everybody, diabetic or not, are well recognized. But people with diabetes have even more reason to get their arms and legs moving, and their hearts pumping. Exercise strengthens the heart, helps control blood-sugar levels and increases circulation to the body's extremities. Exercise can cut the level of harmful blood fats (cholesterol and triglycerides) and increase the level of HDL (the good kind of blood fat that protects against heart disease.) Exercise helps you control your weight, increases your stamina and helps you sleep more soundly.

For diabetics in particular, exercise increases the number of insulin receptors on cell surfaces. This means that insulin can find more places to put glucose, and more glucose can get inside cells, helping to maintain normal blood-sugar levels.

Repetitive movements of the large muscles—arms and legs—are best. This includes walking, jogging, swimming, rowing and bicycling. In order to attain the maximum benefits, you have to exercise regularly—at least three times a week for 20 to 30 minutes.

As a diabetic, if your blood-sugar is out of control, or if you have diabetic eye disease, don't lift weights or do anything else that involves pushing or pulling heavy objects. This kind of exertion raises your blood-sugar levels and blood pressure, and can worsen diabetic eye disease.

One of the best exercises is brisk walking. It's by far the safest, least stressful and most productive of all exercises. It improves the efficiency of every unit of insulin taken in or produced by the body.

> *For diabetics: Don't begin an exercise program without first checking with your doctor. If your diabetes isn't under control or if there are complications, exercise can make it worse.*

Because of the potential for harm as well as good, you should take frequent blood-sugar measurements during the first few weeks of your exercise program. Measure your blood glucose 15-30 minutes before you start exercising, immediately after you stop exercising, and then again several hours after exercising. Record these results in a log, and review them with your doctor.

Here are some additional tips about exercise, eating and diabetes that may be helpful to you.

- If your blood-sugar level is significantly above normal immediately after exercise, reduce or eliminate your pre-exercise snack.

- If, during or shortly after exercise, you tend to suffer from low blood-sugar reactions, be prepared to treat such reactions with simple sugars when they occur. It's a good idea to carry a minimum of 60 grams of simple sugar with you when you exercise.

- Wait at least 1½ hours after you eat a meal before you begin to exercise. That will give your body time to handle the glucose from the foods you've ingested.

- An exercise program enhances the body's ability to normalize blood-sugar over the long term. Don't try to use exercise as the way to immediately lower your blood-sugar level. Remember that if your blood-sugar level is *higher* than normal when you start to exercise, it is likely to *rise*, rather than *fall*, after exercise.

- Don't exercise when you are sick, particularly if you have an infection. Blood-sugar levels are often higher when you are ill, and the stress of exercise can elevate them further.

- Use caution if you exercise before bedtime (to avoid possible low blood-sugar while you are sleeping).

- If you are counting calories, check with your doctor about adjusting your pre-exercise medication dosage (oral or insulin) to lower your risk of exercise-induced hypoglycemia.

(Contributed by Dr. Gilbert Manso)

CHAPTER 3

COPING WITH THE PROBLEM

The Three Stages of Mind

In this book, as in my other books, I try to make it clear that I have not had hypoglycemia, but that I have hypoglycemia—it is a continuing condition.

If you have followed a controlled program for a while, you begin to feel better. Usually this is when you believe that perhaps you don't have hypoglycemia after all. This is what I call Stage 1, the confusion stage. You then decide to eat the sugar you have been craving and perhaps, at first, it doesn't give you much of a problem. But what you don't realize is that the more sugar you eat, the more you will want to eat. So you continue to increase your intake of sugar and you slowly slip back into your old eating habits.

Suddenly, you realize that your are not feeling well, and you begin to have serious doubts. You again start trying to find answers to your health problems. You may seek the advice of a different physician, thinking that surely there must be something else wrong with you. You are now going through Stage 2, the denial stage.

So you may go from doctor to doctor, spending thousands of dollars you may not even have in order to find out what is wrong with you. Surely your problem is more complicated than just hypoglycemia. Sound familiar? Often the more we seek, the more confused we become and the more we deny obvious hypoglycemic symptoms. If we look long enough, we will hear what we want to hear.

You finally find a doctor who tells you that your problem isn't hypoglycemia—it's something else. Then your health really gets bad, because now you aren't even trying to control the amount of sugar in your diet.

In most cases, your health gets so bad that you are forced to consider that you might really be a hypoglycemic. Again, you attempt to give up sugar and you begin to follow a somewhat better nutritional program. You start to feel better and you gradually accept the obvious; you can no longer deny your hypoglycemia symptoms. This is Stage 3, the acceptance stage.

This is when your work begins. You are now ready for the learning process of improving your health. You will learn that you can take charge of your own life; you realize that you can do something about the way you feel.

Unless you find someone who really knows about hypoglycemia, you may never gain enough accurate knowledge of it to maintain yourself in good health.

At some point your doctor may ask if you eat a balanced diet. Since the majority of us aren't really clear on what a balanced diet is, the subject is never fully addressed. When asked about our eating habits, most of us will say, with deep conviction, that we do indeed eat a healthy diet. If asked to define this, however, we are generally at a loss. Most of us aren't aware of the healthiest foods for maximum health, in general, and especially for hypoglycemia and diabetes.

Hopefully, after reading the information in this book, you will understand the dietary steps you will need to take in order to begin a health-giving diet.

Coping With Hypoglycemia and Diabetes

Don't feel guilty about your condition. Sometimes you and I get so tired of being different that we feel guilty for putting our families through what we are going through. We have to look at this in another perspective. If this were our spouse or one of our children, wouldn't we do everything we possibly could to help them to improve their health?

Sometimes the people closest to us don't understand what we are going through. It is sometimes hard for another person to realize that what is happening is very real. After my own decision to change and improve my life, I had to be very strong because I was determined that I was going to feel better. The longer I stayed with my program, the more my health improved,and the more my family realized that I was on the right track. I was becoming my old self again, and they could enjoy being with me again. They realized that there was something to what I was trying to do.

In my lectures I always ask the question "What is the hardest part of staying on a controlled program?" Some of the answers I receive are very surprising. Some feel that my suggestions are too hard to follow, that no one can completely avoid sugar in his/her diet. But I always tell them, YOU MUST! As long as you are getting sugar in your diet, you will never feel any better than you do right now.

One reason why my suggestions are hard to follow may be that some consider this a diet. Most of us think of a diet as a temporary inconvenience, and when it is over we can go back to eating the way we used to. I DO NOT CONSIDER THIS A DIET, I THINK OF THIS AS A WAY OF LIFE.

Perhaps you haven't accepted your condition as the way your life will be from now on. But in order to feel good you will have to make some permanent changes. I realized that if I wanted to feel better, I would have to make some major changes in my life, not just for a little while, but FOREVER.

Accept your condition as a fact you cannot change, and decide to work with your condition instead of ignoring or denying it. The sad part about playing with a diet on an on-off basis is that we not only are quite ill most of the time, but we are courting diabetes. If I have a chance to delay diabetes, why can't I avoid it altogether. Staying on a controlled program will help me avoid diabetes. To me, that is definitely worth the effort.

I had a lady at one of my lectures ask me when she could go back to eating her fast food hamburgers again. When I told her NEVER, I thought she was going to cry. If you are going to stabilize your blood sugar you will have to make up your mind that this is a permanent condition. So what do you do when you want a hamburger? You can't have the fast food delight anymore; it is on white bread made with sugar. The dressing used on the hamburger will also have sugar, the meat will likely have bread crumbs in it, which also have sugar. The catsup will have sugar and in some places the french fries have been sprinkled with a salt/sugar combination to make them more appealing.

You can see how much sugar you can consume before you even get to that little apple pie on the counter.

So what do you do? YOU IMPROVISE! The name of the game is substitution.

Before I became a vegetarian, we had this great little hamburger place with the nicest people and the best hamburgers in town. I knew the owner and I felt sure she would understand my problem and, of course, she did. So I would bring my own bread, my own mayonnaise, and even one cup of whole wheat flour in a Ziploc bag so they could bread my onion rings in the whole wheat flour instead of the white flour they used. This way I didn't feel left out when we went out for hamburgers.

I would not advise anyone to have hamburgers and onion rings every day, and now I would not recommend eating meat or fried foods at all, but at the time it was nice to know that I didn't have to do without a hamburger forever. So you see, where there is a will, there is a way.

Anxiety Attacks and Blood Sugar

If you are unfortunate enough to have these, you know that panic attacks are the most misunderstood of all our problems. You can't explain why you are reacting to a certain situation in totally irrational panic-but you are. I had days when I just wanted to sit in a dark room, curled up in a chair, not wanting to talk to or face anyone. I just wanted to be left alone. Unless you have gone through this, you will never understand how horrible this feeling can be. Your family certainly does not understand, and you begin to believe that you are going crazy.

One of the biggest problems I faced was traveling. Facing a trip of any kind would send me into a panic. There were times I could not even drive across a simple bridge; it was just out of the question. My throat would tighten up; my mouth would get dry; my heart would start pounding; and I would start sweating. I would have to turn back; I could not have driven across that bridge if my life depended on it. I knew, intellectually, that this was completely irrational, but I could not help it.

Then there were times it didn't bother me at all. Now I understand the role my blood-sugar level played with these feelings.

For many years, when I was able to take a long trip, I would get depressed after driving a few hours. I would feel that we were going backward instead of forward and that we would never get there. I had such poor bladder control because of the chronic urethritis that we had to stop every few miles. My family had more patience than I could have dreamed of or wished for. There were times I would start crying for no reason, and we would stop the car and walk around a bit, until I could regain my composure. When I was feeling better, we would continue our trip. By the time we arrived, I would always have a splitting headache and be completely exhausted. I would take my Stanback and Valium and lie down for an hour or so. My doctor simply ignored any questions I had about this problem. Since he didn't have an explanation for these attacks, as far as he was concerned they didn't exist.

I have seen several documentaries done on panic or anxiety attacks, and each time I notice there is never, at any time, any mention of the possibility that a drop in blood sugar levels could be a cause of this problem. The patients are given drugs and undergoes psychiatric care, but they are never even questioned about their nutritional habits.

I am not saying that biofeedback or psychiatric care is not an important part of learning how to deal with the situation; in many cases these have a very important role in a patient's complete recovery. What I am suggesting is that no matter what type of counseling one may have, unless the blood sugar is controlled, these attacks will continue to occur. You may know better how to deal with the attacks to some extent, but you also know that the attacks are still happening to you.

Please understand that I am not saying I have the complete answer to this problem. What I am saying is that the nutrition and the natural approach can only help the situation, be it medical or psychological. I had a young lady call me late one night in a total panic. She was so upset that it took me a while to calm her down, to make her understand, to put the phone down and get herself a piece of cheese. After about ten minutes, she was calm enough to think straight. She told me that the piece of cheese had done more for her than all the years of psychiatric care had ever done.

One young man admitted to me that after all the years of biofeedback and psychiatric care, he was still having these attacks. Through counseling sessions, he was better informed as to how to handle them, but nonetheless, they were still happening. Even though his doctors knew of his history of hypoglycemia, they had never considered that it might be a contributing factor in his attacks. From my own experience I have found that I was much better off taking a B-complex vitamin and a calcium supplement for my nerves than a valium or other drug. Take it from someone who has had to kick her dependency to valium—it isn't easy. It took me a good six months before I was able to get off that drug. I don't believe I could have done it without the aid of vitamin supplements. Only the natural approach gets the results that can benefit your body on a lasting basis.

I now travel anywhere without even a thought that I cannot do it. I make several out-of-town trips each year, lecturing to different hypoglycemic groups and organizations. A few years ago this would have been out of the question for me. Even driving on the interstate was at one time impossible; now on many occasions I travel alone without fear or panic. How wonderful it is to feel free! Get that blood sugar under control, and you too can live a life free from fear and uncertainty.

Believe me, it feels great!

CHAPTER 4

Developing An
Appropriate Lifestyle

Starting a Diet

It is important to keep in mind that moderation is the key to your recovery. When you first start on the program, you may not be able to tolerate some of the higher carbohydrate foods. As your health improves, your body will be able to handle these foods. If you are a diabetic, you may not be able to tolerate fruits at all. We are all individuals. You have to find out what will work for you. Start slowly, give your body time to heal.

Because we have to eat so often, eating can sometimes become boring. We all get tired of the same old foods. Psychologically, we need a boost. I also believe that we all have a need to have something that tastes sweet every now and then. You would never think of giving a dinner party without serving a dessert or of going through the holidays without something sweet. No one likes the idea of being different, so being able to entertain or go through the holidays like everyone else is very important.

As free adults, we have the God-given right to take charge of our own bodies. We are responsible for our own health—not our doctor, or our family—only us. It is time we face our problems and realize that unless we take measures to correct our nutritional habits, we will not improve our health.

Sometimes people tell me that they don't have enough willpower to stick to my nutritional suggestions. I don't think it takes willpower; I think it takes common sense. Even an animal will not continue doing something that he knows will hurt him. He may do it twice, but I bet you he won't do it the third time. Eating the right foods and staying away from white flour and sugar isn't hard when you know the payoff is feeling good. It has now been many years since I have had refined sugar. I would not give up feeling good for anything. If I want a food bad enough, I will turn it around and make it without sugar so it won't make me ill.

Coping with Stress

Stress can have the most devastating effect on us. As hypoglycemics or diabetics, we are not able to handle stress well. It can literally wipe us out. We need to take life one day at a time and pace ourselves so that we do not overdo.

Stress is a way of life. Let's face it, even getting out of bed in the morning or opening our mail can result in a stressful situation. If the body isn't healthy, we can't deal with that stress. We need to minimize the stress in our lives whenever possible, but also remember that it will always be a part of our lives. Only when the body is healthy, can we cope with whatever life demands of us.

Special Situations
(Eating Out, Vacations, Holidays)

Keep in mind that your hypoglycemia or diabetes NEVER TAKES A VACATION! Just because you are away from home on a trip is no reason to have sugar and junk. How much more enjoyable your trip will be if your energy level is the way it should be, or if you don't have to put up with a headache the whole trip. While you are traveling, EAT! Bring a tote bag stocked with fruits, cheese and nuts; perhaps a thermos containing a protein drink. Eat often—you need to keep up your energy.

Traveling is very stressful. I have found that increasing my Vitamin B-Complex, and Vitamin C is helpful. If you stop at a restaurant, be sure the food you order doesn't have sugar. Eating out can sometimes be a problem. At first you may feel that you will never enjoy an evening out again. NOT SO! Extra precautions have to be taken, but you will find that going out to dinner can be just as enjoyable as it always was. Don't make eating out a habit, because nutrition suffers somewhat when you eat out.

When you are getting ready to eat out, always bring your own salad dressing. Tupperware makes a 2 oz. midget container that comes in very handy. It holds just enough dressing for one salad and fits nicely in your handbag or pocket.

If you must eat bread with your restaurant meal, the R. W. Knudsen Sourdough Bread Chips are excellent. Other whole wheat crackers from your health food stores are also okay. Place a handful in a Ziploc bag and just bring them out when you are ready for your salad. You may want to bring enough for everyone at the table because they are so good that everyone will end up eating your bread chips instead of those awful white crackers that are on the table.

Always ask the waitress if what you are ordering has sugar. Don't ask casually, which invites the waitress to say, equally casually, "Gee, I don't think so." Make sure she knows, and if she doesn't know, ask her to check with the chef. Most restaurants are very helpful, and will go out of their way to satisfy you. I have even gone into the kitchen and talked to the chef myself about a special dish I wanted to order.

If you want to order something like fried fish, ask them to use cornmeal instead of white flour to bread the fish. Cornmeal is a complex carbohydrate and can be tolerated much better than the white flour. Always be sure that the dish is not pre-breaded, because that will always have sugar in it.

Be careful of ordering foods that have tomato sauce in them unless you are sure about the kind of tomatoes used. Most canned tomatoes will have sugar in them. If the establishment isn't helpful to your needs, get up and go somewhere else. A bit of awkwardness or some inconvenience is a small price to pay for feeling healthy.

For most of us the holiday season is the hardest time to do without sugar. We feel deprived because we can't have all the good tasting sweets we used to have. We can't stand being deprived, so we give in. You should just realize that your health problems NEVER TAKE A HOLI-DAY! Your body doesn't know this is a special occasion and to think that it will not react to your indulgence is pure folly. For a moment's pleasure, it can take you weeks, even months, for your body to recuperate from your binge.

I have provided several holiday recipes which will help you get through the season in good health. Just because you can't have sugars is no reason that you can't have sweets. Your holiday will be much more enjoyable if you feel good and have the energy to do all you need to do for yourself and your family. I dare say I have never had anyone turn down a meal at my house, especially during the holidays. You don't have to tell anyone that the food he/she is about to eat doesn't have sugar. You can fix a delicious meal without a grain of sugar.

Section II

The Program

CHAPTER 5

Nutrition and Weight Maintenance

Nutritional Suggestions to Rebuild Your Health

1. Eliminate sugar and white flour completely from your diet. Think of them as poison to your body because that is what they are. Arsenic is a poison, and you wouldn't eat it because you know it will eventually kill you. Put your sugar bowl in the same category as that bottle of arsenic, and you won't have any trouble staying away from these products or anything made with them.

2. Eat six to eight times a day. Eating frequent small meals will help you to stabilize your blood sugar. You are not overtaxing your digestive system when you eat small meals. The food you eat will digest slowly, giving your body a constant supply of energy. The food you eat will be used for energy, not stored into fat, and you will be much more able to control your blood sugar and your weight.

3. Eat more complex carbohydrates instead of animal protein. Don't forget that nuts, seeds, and beans are also excellent sources of protein, and in moderation should cause no problems. Your complex carbohydrates are any whole grains, fresh fruits, vegetables, legumes, and tubers such as potatoes and taro.

4. At least once a day have a raw vegetable/fruit plate, with any available fresh vegetables and fruits. Raw vegetables and fruits give your body necessary bulk and fiber to keep the colon healthy and aid in the elimination process.

5. Fruit juices, if used, should be in moderation. Dilute them half and half with water. Even if the juice has no sugar added, it is a much too concentrated natural sugar to have at one time and your body cannot handle it. I prefer to squeeze my own juice. It is healthier and tastier, but I still add extra water to it. Although fresh-squeezed does give you some of the pulp from the fruit, it is still too much sugar for your body to handle at one time.

6. Honey is allowed occasionally in small amounts. Use only 1/2 teaspoon at a time, and very rarely. Do not use it until after your blood sugar has been stable for some time.

7. If you are out for a while, something may delay you and you will need a pickup. Have food with you at all times. Carry nuts or seeds in your handbag or pocket.

8. I suggest you purchase a small carbohydrate counter from your health food store or local bookstore. I found this very helpful in learning which foods have the most carbohydrates.

9. When you are eating carbohydrates, try to always eat some protein as well. Protein slows down the metabolism of carbohydrates into glucose and helps to stabilize your blood sugar. Also, listen to your body and let it tell you what your carbohydrate limit should be.

10. On days when you are under extra stress, you may find that you may have to eat more often. Stress can set you back almost as much as eating sugar. It will be helpful for you to take a few precautions on the days that you know will be extra stressful or demanding. I have found that taking extra vitamin supplements prior to whatever stress I am about to face can make a big difference in how I cope. B Complex vitamins, in particular, help to smooth the metabolism of carbohydrates that you've consumed.

11. If you have enjoyed a special type of food that is not allowed in your diet, find a pleasing substitute. Don't continue to feel deprived, because if you feel deprived you will cheat, and if you cheat you are only cheating yourself. If you eat sugar, either accidentally or intentionally, it will be absorbed into your bloodstream, causing the pancreas to release high insulin levels that will produce symptoms of hypoglycemia. It is important to have a protein snack every two hours to help counteract the effect of this high insulin release. When you have a frequent protein snack, you will find that you will not have as much trouble with the low periods which follow high insulin release. Taking extra B-Complex vitamins will also help during this time. Within a day or so you can go back to your regular schedule.

12. Most hypoglycemics and diabetics suffer from some form of allergy. You will find most of the recipes in this book are made with whole wheat flour. Those of you with an allergy to wheat may need to substitute some other kind of whole grain you can tolerate. In many cases, even with severe allergies, getting on the nutritional foods and supplements that we recommend will lessen your allergic reaction a great deal, and in time foods you may not have been able to tolerate in the past won't bother you. You will be building your body's own immune system and the results are amazing. Give your body the right tools and in many cases it will heal itself.

13. If you feel hypoglycemia symptoms coming on, you may want to use a "quick fix," using a protein snack plus four times your usual B-Complex vitamin dosage (of the dosage you normally take). This is especially helpful if you have eaten sugar and find that your blood sugar is very unstable.

14. If you wake up during the night and have trouble going back to sleep, don't just toss and turn. You need to get up and have a snack. One of the reasons you can't get back to sleep is that your blood sugar is too low. I have found that taking 1000 mgs. of magnesium along with a snack is much better than taking a sleeping pill.

15. If you have "restless legs syndrome" during the night, it may be an indication that your blood sugar is too low. Your muscles need a certain amount of glucose in order to function, and when your blood sugar level is too low, your muscles are actually screaming for energy. Again, I recommend you eat a little food. This will help raise that blood sugar and keep it up. Taking 400 to 800 IU's of Vitamin E during the day is also a big help.

16. The high fiber diet that is so beneficial for hypoglycemics and diabetics causes some changes in the way some vitamins and minerals are absorbed—calcium, in particular. Since a high fiber meal can interfere with the absorption of calcium, I recommend you take your calcium and other minerals either thirty minutes before your high fiber meal, or an hour after. It is also important to take a part of your calcium supplement before bedtime, and if possible, with a digestive aid ("Beta-Gest" or an equivalent hydrochloric acid supplement). This way you are assured of the highest absorption. Calcium aids sleep and rest throughout the night. It is often called "nature's tranquilizer."

17. Smoking. There is no way you will be able to completely control your blood sugar if you smoke. Cigarettes can cause your blood sugar to take a sudden rise with the first puff and just as rapid a drop after the cigarette is out. This could explain the habit of chain smoking. The craving for another cigarette could really be a craving to replenish the lowered blood-sugar level.

18. Candy Bars. If your weakness is a candy bar, try a fruit juice sweetened candy bar instead, or a Carafection Bar from your health food store. It is delicious and a complex carbohydrate, so you are able to tolerate these in small amounts. If you are a diabetic, be careful not to have these too often. If you have a problem controlling your blood sugar, stay away from these.

    I don't advise having "candy" often, but every now and then, it is nice to think you can be like everyone else. If you have a weight problem, be sure you count the calories in the candy in with your allowed caloric intake for the day.

19. Bread Crumbs. Almost all commercial bread and all commercial bread crumbs have sugar in them. I tried making bread crumbs from homemade whole wheat bread, but it was too coarse. I now use whole grain wheat cereal. I put it in the blender and get fine bread crumbs. Add a few spices and you have Italian bread crumbs, a healthy alternative.

20. Bread. I don't know about you, but I used to have a devil of a time getting my dough to rise. After several disastrous attempts, I decided to place my dough in the oven with the door slightly ajar. This is done the first time you allow the dough to rise. Set the temperature on the lowest keep-warm setting. The results are fascinating, beautiful dough doubled in size in one hour. Remember,

the softer your dough is the second time you knead it, the softer your bread will be.

21. Gravies. To thicken gravies, don't use cornstarch, which is quickly converted to glucose in your body. Use one tablespoon of whole wheat flour instead. It does a great job of thickening the gravy and is better tolerated than cornstarch.

22. Alcohol of any kind is out because alcohol is even more harmful than sugar. On the studies done on alcoholism, it has been found that alcoholics are almost always hypoglycemics as well. When they were placed on a hypoglycemia control program, the need for alcohol was often gone. It is believed by some experts that an alcoholic is really craving the sugar that is in the alcohol, not the alcohol itself. It was discovered that when alcoholics were put on a hypoglycemia control program, the number who returned to drinking was remarkably low compared to the group treated only for psychiatric problems. It is sad that some doctors still believe that psychiatric care is the only important form of treatment and neglect nutrition. How much more effective the AA programs would be if they served a nutritious snack instead of the coffee and donuts they often serve. I have often heard it said that you can take an alcoholic off the alcohol, but can't take away his sweets. Can't we realize that hypoglycemia is at the root of the problem?

At a party, instead of drinking wine, which contains sugar in addition to the alcohol, drink Club Soda with a twist of lemon or lime. Bring your own bottle if necessary. You can get it at any grocery store. Drink it from an attractive wine glass. It tastes great and you won't feel left out without a drink in your hand.

23. You should stay away from caffeine as if it were sugar. Caffeine stimulates the adrenal glands, causing a high insulin release from the pancreas. It is therefore impossible to control the blood sugar level if you drink caffeine. Some coffees and teas are decaffeinated by a process that uses toxic chemicals, and trace amounts of these chemicals have been found in the finished products. Other decaffeinated products use only natural substances for decaffeination. So if you need to drink coffee or nonherbal tea, make sure the label on the container says "naturally decaffeinated"

There are many delicious herbal teas on the market which serve as an excellent substitute. Your health food stores will also have coffee substitutes, and although they do not have the exact taste of coffee, they are quite tasty.

24. Many hypoglycemics are also hypothyroid (low thyroid output). I suggest you take your basal temperature (temperature taken at rest) for three days in a row. If your temperature is lower than 97.8 degrees, this could be an indication that your thyroid could use a little help. You will want to discuss this with your doctor. He may recommend a thyroid medication, or a thyroid stimulator. If you are a diabetic, taking a thyroid medication will help protect you against some of the degenerative problems you are facing.

25. Daily exercise is most important. Your blood sugar is stabilized while you are exercising and this plays a major role in controlling it. Clinical tests have proven that your body undergoes a complete metabolic change with daily exercise. In time you will find you will be better able to control your hypoglycemia or diabetes. Even the symptoms of depression and fatigue will be lessened. High blood pressure and high triglycerides are also lowered with regular exercise. Note Dr. Manso's information on exercise for the diabetic patient.

    Even if you feel you don't have the energy, it is very important that you initiate some type of exercise program. As soon as you do, your energy level will begin to pick up.

26. Remember that too much of anything can be harmful. No matter how good something may be, anything can be overdone. Moderation is the key to everything.

Your body didn't get in this shape overnight. It will take a while before it will be completely healthy again. Give your body time to heal itself.

A Nutritional Summary

- Do not have sugar, white flour, white rice, caffeine or alcohol in any way. No matter how small the amount it will throw your blood sugar off.

- Eat every two hours, only in small amounts, and only vegetables, complex carbohydrates and high quality (complete) proteins.

- Throughout the day, always back up your high complex carbohydrate diet with protein. This can be your protein drink, or other high quality, complete protein foods.

- Find the highest quality vitamin/mineral supplement on the market and take it regularly.

- Exercise every day.

There is never just one thing you need to do to rebuild your health. It is a combination of efforts that will mean success or failure. Give your body time to heal. Give our program 100% and you will see that it will work. Don't cheat. You can't give it 50% and expect 100% results. Life is too short to spend it feeling bad. Do something about your condition now. You will never regret it.

For the Junk Food Junkie

I confess that I was a "Junk Food Junkie." Had I not been, I would not have had these problems with my health. We can't put garbage into our bodies day after day, year after year, and expect to enjoy a long, healthy, productive life. Our bodies can only handle so much sugar, preservatives, dyes, and carcinogens. Eventually we'll have to pay the price of ill health; it will catch up with us.

Several years ago, I realized that if I were ever to regain my health, major changes were required in both my nutritional habits and in the way I viewed my life. Life is a learning experience, and nutritional knowledge doesn't happen overnight. We need to take it one day at a time. I have no illusions that everyone reading this book will empty their pantries of all unhealthy foods. I only hope to make you aware that changes are necessary if you are to achieve better health. It is important that we begin to make healthier food choices. When I started on my road to better health, I concentrated only on eliminating sugars. As I began to understand what was involved in living a healthier life, I realized it was much more complicated than that.

Most of us need some specific reason to even consider making major dietary changes in our lives. It doesn't matter what the problems are; if they're not severe enough to seek medical advise, we do not pay attention. Even then, we choose to ignore the problem, fooling ourselves that it will go away. It's time we take charge of our own lives. We, and no one else, are responsible for our own health. It isn't the easy way, but it's the only way.

Most of the food producers expect us to take the easy way out when it comes to preparing our foods. Most of us lead busy lives. We believe that we don't have the time it takes to prepare a healthy meal. We settle for the fast foods, seldom giving nutrition a thought. Some people believe that they can't afford to eat healthily. In reality, it costs less to eat a healthy meal than it would cost for us to settle for that fast food meal.

Others believe that they can't give up the sweets. One of the hardest things to convince anyone of is that if they give up the sugars, they won't crave them anymore. I know it is hard to believe, when you would probably be willing to KILL for that candy bar. But believe me, once you get the sugar out of your system and your blood sugar is under control, you will not crave the sugars anymore. I strongly believe that we need to get away from having something that tastes sweet everyday, even if it doesn't have real sugar in it. I don't believe that we need to eat a dessert everyday. Now and then indulge yourself, have that special treat, but make it without the sugar. To enjoy something that tastes sweet every now and then, makes us feel that we are not so different after all, that we are almost like everyone else.

We, too, can enjoy something sinful now and then and get away with it, if we make it without the sugar. When you feel that you are losing control, make it a sugar-free treat. By doing it this way, you won't have to feel guilty or pay the price for your weakness.

In order to help facilitate the need for sweets, I have compiled a list of some HEALTHY JUNK FOOD you can find at any health food store. Please remember that these are to be used sparingly.

SUPPLIER CODE:

R. W. Knudsen — — — — — — —KND
Barbara's Bakery   — — — — — —BBK
Little Bear Trading Co.   — — — —LBT
Nature's Warehouse, INC.   — — —NW
Tree of Life — — — — — — — — —TL
West Brae, INC. — — — — — — —WB

Cookies (BBK)
  Creme Vanilla
  Creme Fudge
  Fruit & Nut
  Oatmeal Raisin
  Almond
  Peanut Butter
  Coconut
  Animal Cookies/Vanilla
  Date/Walnut
  Butter Vanilla
  Carob Snap
  Oatmeal Snap
  Lemon Snap
  Peanut Butter Snap
  Carob Coated Peanuts

Granola Bars (BBK)
  Cinnamon/Oat
  Cocoa/Almond
  Peanut Butter

Candies (NW)
  Animal Cookies/Cinnamon
  No-How Peanut Butter
  Nougat Bar
  Nut-Wit, Carob, Caramel
  Peanut Bar
  Non-Stop Carob, Coconut
  Caramel Bar

Carafection (TL)
  Carob-Coated Almonds
  Carob-Coated Raisins

Chips & Crackers
  Sourdough Bread Chips (KND)
  Whole Wheat Bagel Chips (KND)
  Corn Chips (BBK)
  Potato Chips (BBK)
  Cheese Puffs (BBK)
  Yogurt & Onion Potato Chips (BBK)
  Bearito Corn Chips (LBT)
  Blue Corn Chips (LBT)
  Nacho Blue Corn Chips (LBT)
  Blue Bearitos (LBT)
  Bearitos (LBT)
  Brown Rice Snaps (WB)
  Taco Shells (LBT)
  Tostada Shells (LBT)
  Pepper Crispbread (BBK)
  Sesame Crispbread (BBK)
  Sesame Brown Rice Snaps (WB)

---

* All of these products are made without any refined sugars, and contain NO hydrogenated oils or preservatives.

Vegetarianism

There are various reasons why some of us choose to give up eating meat. I used to think vegetarians were people with weird thoughts about religion and other things. Now that I am one, I understand a little more about why some people choose to give up meat in their daily diet.

I thoroughly enjoyed eating meat, especially red meat. Although I knew I shouldn't eat red meat as often as I did, I didn't really know how to give it up. We develop our eating habits very early in life, and like my mother and grandmother before her, I planned my meal around my meat dish. Without the meat, I really didn't know what to serve. To be honest, I probably would never have given up meat had it not been for writing this book. Often, during the first few months of my new program, I would recall Dr. Manso's words, "If it doesn't grow on a tree or bush, you can't have it." So it was an adjustment to say the least.

Since I am not one to say one thing and do another, I felt I had no choice but to at least give it an honest effort and try. Now, as with so many other changes in my life, it is no longer an effort, but has become a way of life.

Many of us do not understand what being a vegetarian means. Availability and tradition play an important role in determining the types of foods we eat. Whichever foods we may choose to eat, there are certain nutritional needs we must meet in order to maintain a healthy active life. The following are the different categories of practicing vegetarianism.

Vegan Vegetarians: Individuals who abstain from all forms of animal foods, including red meat, poultry, fish or seafood, eggs and dairy products.

Lacto-Ovo Vegetarians: Individuals whose consumption of animal products includes only milk and eggs.

Lacto Vegetarians: Individuals who consume milk and milk products, but no other animal products.

Ovo Vegetarians: Individuals who consume eggs, but no other animal products.

Semi-Vegetarians: Individuals who may use certain animal products if they are prepared in a particular way or under certain conditions.

People are turning to vegetarianism more and more as a means of achieving better health. It is one of the most effective means of treating and controlling high blood pressure, high cholesterol, and obesity. You may ask, if it is that simple, why aren't more of us vegetarians? The problem is that it isn't that simple. Our eating habits are the hardest of all habits to change. To become a vegetarian means drastic measures have to be taken to change those eating habits. When drastic measures are necessary to correct ill health, not everyone is prepared to take such action. Even when facing death, some of us are not able to make the commitment to give up some of our favorite foods, though we know these foods are the reason for our illness. The old saying, "we dig our graves with our forks," has never been truer.

It isn't always easy to consume a balanced intake of the essential nutrients when one is practicing vegetarianism. Adequate protein intake is especially critical for those of us who are hypoglycemics and diabetics. It is a fact that plant products can be limited in some of the essential proteins. Therefore, it is important that one fully understand what is involved in being a vegetarian.

Soy protein is an excellent choice as a vegetable protein source. Some vegetable proteins, such as legumes, lack in certain essential amino acids and are known as incomplete proteins. But consumed together with whole grains, they form a complete protein. They should be eaten within twenty minutes of each other or, even better, at the same time. For example, red beans with cornbread, or red beans and brown rice make a complete, high quality protein source. In general, any bean eaten together with any grain make a complete protein.

The vegetarian must become well informed about the best sources of nutrients. He should select and consume foods on the basis of providing a complete and balanced intake of nutrients. The information provided in the following chapter will help you in making the proper food choices.

CHAPTER 6

THE DO's AND DON'T's OF EATING

How to Eat

1. Eat only when hungry.

2. Eat small meals several times a day.

3. Eat slowly in a relaxed, unhurried atmosphere.

4. When protein rich foods are eaten with other foods, eat the protein foods first.

5. Unless you are underweight, practice systematic "under-eating"—eating less than you feel you need.

6. Eat more raw fresh vegetables and fruits. If you do cook your vegetables, cook only slightly or lightly steam.

7. Do not drink with your meals. You need the HCL which is present in your stomach to digest your foods.

8. Drink clean healthy water. If you do not have a water purifying system, use bottled spring water. Use it for drinking, cooking, ice cubes, etc.

Foods That Are Allowed

Carbohydrates:

Whole Grain Bread (homemade or health food store)
Oat flour
Oatmeal (cooked or uncooked), oat bran
Soy grits(cooked or uncooked)
Wheat germ
Whole wheat flour , wheat bran
Any whole grains, such as corn, barley, millet, wild rice, etc.
Noodles, spaghetti and other pasta (Jerusalem artichoke, soy semolina, vegetable semolina, and whole wheat spaghetti, all found in health food stores).
Brown rice
Potatoes
Sweet potatoes
Ezekiel sprouted grain bread (from health food stores)
Whole grain cereals without sugar
Vegetables
Fruits

Condiments & Seasonings:

Prepared mustard (yellow or brown)
Kikkomon Soy Sauce
Herbs (marjoram, oregano, basil, chervil, thyme, parsley, bay leaves, etc.)
Spices (pepper, cloves, cinnamon, paprika, ginger, curry, chili powder, etc.)
Salt (plain or sea salt,)
Onion and onion powder
Onion flakes
Garlic, fresh or powder
Seeds (mustard, caraway, sesame, poppy)
Dry mustard
Celery salt
Dehydrated lemon peel and orange peel
Sugarless seasoning mixtures
Paul Newman Italian Salad Dressing
Flavorings or Extracts (Make sure that vanilla or any other flavoring DO NOT contain sugar in any form. I prefer to purchase these from health food stores in the pure form. They are a little more expensive, but well worth the little extra you may pay.)

Juices & Beverages:

**R. W. Knudsen Brands of Juices & Sodas
Fruit juices (diluted half & half with water)
Ciders
Sparkling juices
Tropical punches
Very Veggie
Vita Juice
Black Cherry Spritzer
Cranberry Spritzer
Grape Spritzer
Lemon Lime Spritzer
Mandarin Orange/Lime Spritzer
Peach Spritzer
Red Raspberry Spritzer
Strawberry Spritzer
Passion Fruit Spritzer
Tangerine Spritzer
Boysenberry Spritzer
Seltzer club sodas
Herb teas
Milk
Vita Soy
Eden Soy
Tomato juices
V-8 juice
Perrier
Dacopa (coffee substitute from health food stores)
Cafix (coffee substitute from health food stores)

Please remember that all fruit juices and sodas should be diluted half & half with water or Perrier and used sparingly. Diabetics are not allowed fruit juices as a general rule.

Sweeteners:

Devan Sweet — Devansoy Farms brand (from health food stores)
Dr. Bronner's barley malt sweetener
Liquid barley malt (from health food stores)
Rice Syrup (Chico-San Yinnies brand from health food store)
Rice Syrup (Sweet Cloud brand from health food store)
Fruit Juice Sweeteners (Wax Brand and natural fruit juice concentrate from health food store)
Dates (no-sugar kind from health food store or Dromedary brand NATURAL FRUIT ONLY in your grocery store)

Syrups allowed:
R. W. Knudsen Brands:
Blueberry syrup
Boysenberry syrup
Raspberry syrup
Strawberry syrup or pourable strawberry topping

Jellies & Jams allowed:
West Brae Brands:
Strawberry Conserves
Grape Conserves
Marmalade
Orange
All jelly & jam conserves WITHOUT SUGAR from grocery stores

The barley malts, rice syrups, & fruit sweeteners are tolerated in small amounts. These products do not call on a high insulin release from the pancreas into the bloodstream as sugars do.

Oils:
Olive oil (the best choice)
Canola oil (by Spectrum Naturals)
Peanut oil
Oleic Safflower oil
Butter
Pam

Proteins:
Raw nuts and seeds
Whole grains
Fresh vegetables
Fresh fruits
Yogurt(plain)
Kefir
Soy foods
Tofu
Buttermilk

**eat only fresh foods

If you must eat animal protein:
    1st choice: Fish with fins and scales
    2nd choice: Eggs
    3rd choice: Poultry
    4th choice: White cheese
    5th choice: Lamb

Cereals:
    Nabisco Cream of Wheat
    Quaker Old Fashioned Oats
    Uncle Sam Natural Cereal
    Kellogg's Nutri-Grain Cereal
    Nabisco Shredded Wheat
    Nabisco Toasted Wheat & Raisins
    Post Grape Nuts & Raisins
    Post Grape Nuts
    Health Valley Sprouts 7
    Health Valley Bran Cereal
    Health Valley Wheat Germ
    Health Valley Amaranth
    ConAgri Cream of Rye
    Oat Bran Cereal
    Rice Cream Cereal
    Seven Grain Cereal

Shopping list for Complex Carbohydrates:

Vegetables:	Fruits:	Grains & Legumes:
Artichokes	Apples	Barley
Asparagus	Apricots	Beans (dried)
Avocados	Bananas	Brown rice
Beets	Blackberries	Corn
Bean sprouts	Blueberries	Couscous
Broccoli	Cantaloupe	Cracked wheat
Brussels sprouts	Cherries	Garbanzo(chick peas)
Cabbage	Dates	Lentils
Carrots	Figs	Millet
Celery	Grapes	Oats
Chard	Grapefruit	Tabouli
Chinese cabbage	Honeydew melon	Wild rice
Collard greens	Muskmelon	
Cucumbers	Oranges	

Vegetables:	Fruits:	Grains & Legumes:
Dandelion greens	Peaches	
Eggplant	Pears	
Garlic	Pineapple	
Greens (Beet)	Plums	
Greens (Mustard)	Prunes	
Horseradish	Raspberries	
Kohlrabi	Strawberries	
Leeks	Tangerines	
Lettuce	Watermelon	
Okra		
Olives (ripe)		
Onions		
Peas		
Peppers		
Parsnips		
Potatoes		
Pumpkin		
Rutabagas		
String beans		
Summer squash		
Tomatoes		
Turnips		
Turnip greens		
Watercress		
Winter squash		
Yellow squash		

Pastas:

DeBoles Jerusalem Artichoke Pastas
Lasagna-Semolina
Lasagna-Whole Wheat
Noodles-Semolina

What Is Not Allowed in Your Diet

Canned vegetables containing sugar
Frozen vegetables in sauces
All processed meats: bacon, ham, sausage, etc.

Fats:
    Butter whipped in honey
    Imitation dairy products for coffee
    Mayonnaise (unless specified sugarless)
    Prepared salad dressings (unless specified sugarless)

Condiments & Seasonings:
    Most combination herb seasonings
    Meatloaf seasonings
    Gravy mixes
    Chili sauce
    Ketchup
    Marinades
    Smoke flavorings
    Mayonnaise & mayonnaise salad dressings
    Most soy sauces
    Steak sauces
    Cocktail sauces for seafood
    Seasoned salts containing sugar (lemon salt, butter flavored salt)
    Butter buds
    Potato buds
    Bottled salad dressings (unless specified sugar-free)
    Barbecue sauce
    Meat tenderizers
    Prepared dips
    Worcestershire sauce
    Bouillon cubes and packets

Beverages:
    Wine
    Beer
    Hard liquor
    Cordials
    Any other alcoholic beverages
    Cooking wine in food
    All colas, diet colas, or other sodas, except for those listed.
        Lemonade(with sugar)
    Grape juice
    Tea with caffeine
    Instant tea mix

Punch
Ovaltine
Chocolate milk
Hot chocolate
Orange breakfast drinks
Coffee (with caffeine)
Decaffeinated coffee and tea (These have other chemicals besides caffeine which can stimulate high insulin release.)

Artificial Sweeteners:

Weight Watchers brand
Sweeta
Sweet & Low
Sweet One
Most sprinkle-type sweeteners
Equal packages(contains sugar)
Any other sweetener containing sugar in any form.

Avoid sugar in any form—These are the different names to watch out for:

Honey	Maple syrup
Syrup	Maple sugar
Corn syrup	Heavy syrup
Molasses	Invert sugar
Raw sugar	Refined sugar
Cane sugar	Confectioner's sugar
Brown sugar	Sucrose
Mannitol	Glucose
Sorbitol	Fructose
Dextrose	Maltose, malt
Corn syrup solids	Sorghum syrup
Nutritive sweeteners	Sorghum
Caramels	Turbinado sugar
High corn syrup	

Dextrins and Maltodextrins are derivatives of starch, and starch is quickly converted into sugar in the body. If eaten in large amounts, these kinds of starch can give you problems. Where they are included in puddings, eat in moderation because other kinds of starches are also added.

Basic Rules for Foods to Avoid

* Enriched refined flours
* Refined sugars
* Foods containing added vegetables oils
* Foods containing or cooked in lard.
* Processed foods (they are full of chemicals)
* Cola drinks
* Chocolate
* Alcohol
* Candy
* Ice Cream
* Hamburgers
* Processed cheeses
* Beef
* Pork
* Pizza
* All frozen dinners
* Processed meats
* Most canned foods
* Caffeinated beverages
* Tea
* Coffee
* Decaffeinated coffee (except naturally-decaffeinated)
* Soft drinks
* Root beers
* Juice drinks
* Gatorade
* Kool-aid
* Commercially prepared bouillon
* Commercial salad dressings
* Catsup
* Hot dogs
* Hydrogenated oils
* Margarine

Caffeine and anything made with it:

Causes breast tenderness, increases anxiety, irritability, and mood swings. Also depletes the body of the B vitamins thus interfering with carbohydrate metabolism.

Soft drinks and anything made with them:

All have artificial sweeteners and artificial flavorings as well as phosphoric, citric, and other strong acids added to sugar-free drinks. These are harmful and should be avoided.

Chocolate and anything made with it:

Worsens mood swings, increases irritability, intensifies sugar craving, causes weight gain, increases the body's need for B-Complex vitamins, and causes breast tenderness because it contains caffeine.

Sugar and anything made with it:

Depletes the body of B vitamins and minerals. Calls on a high insulin release from the pancreas into the bloodstream. It is HAZARDOUS TO YOUR HEALTH.

Alcohol and anything made with it:

Depletes the body of all the vitamins, especially the B vitamins, and all minerals. It disrupts carbohydrate metabolism, is toxic to the liver, and will impair the liver functions. It kills brain cells by the millions and causes the destruction of cells throughout the body. It also impairs thinking, causes extreme personality changes, and increases irritability.

Beef and Pork and anything made with them:

They are high in fat which can compromise liver efficiency. Most contain synthetic hormones, antibiotics, and other chemicals which impair liver functions. Bacon and ham contain nitrites which are carcinogens (cancer causing agents.)

Dairy Products:

Many people are "Milk intolerant." They lack the necessary enzymes to digest milk products, or they are allergic to milk. In both instances, milk products produce gas and digestive problems. Stay away from dairy products. They are mucus producing, constipating, and generally unhealthy.

Salt and high sodium foods:

Too much salt can worsen fluid retention, bloating, breast tenderness. Most processed foods contain lots of salt and are nothing but chemical-loaded garbage.

All commercial dressings and processed foods and anything made with them:

They contain chemicals toxic to the body in varying degrees. These additives are responsible for ailments ranging from hyperactivity in children to heart disease and cancer.

Eat only small amounts of oranges, grapefruit, papaya, pineapple, tomatoes, potatoes, eggplant, and spinach.

These foods are high in simple sugars and have high acid content.

Avoid all processed, canned, refined, and other denatured super-market foods.

Additives and Medications

Additives to Avoid:
* BHA and BHT
* Dyes
* Bleaches
* Emulsifiers
* Amino-oxidants
* Preservatives
* Artificial flavors
* Flavor Enhancers, such as Monosodium Glutamate (MSG)
* Buffers
* Acidifiers
* Extenders
* Disinfectants
* Defoliants
* Fungicides
* Neutralizers
* Anti-Caking and Anti-Foaming agents (these contain aluminum)
* Conditioners
* Dough Conditioners
* Curers
* Hydrolyzers
* Maturers
* Fortifiers
* Antibiotics
* Arsenic

* Artificial Sex Hormones
* Hydrogenated Oils
* Pesticides
* Sugars

Medications Not Recommended:

Aspirin containing caffeine
Anacin
Empirin
APC
Bromo Seltzer Tablets
4-Way Cold Tablets
Trigesin
Fiorinal
NoDoz/Vivarin
Midol
B C Tablets
Cough drops
NyQuil

The following was collected from a local pharmacy to give you additional information on cold and sinus medications. Be careful of all cough medicines containing alcohol, honey or sugar syrup, and codeine. Also, antihistamines can play havoc with your blood sugar.

Sugar Free Cough/Cold Preparations (most contain alcohol):

CODES:

RX—By prescription only
OTC—Over the counter
CII—Controlled, Class two (must sign for)
CIII—Controlled, Class three (must sign for)
CIV—Controlled, Class four (must sign for)
  * Medications that are alcohol free and sugar free.
  ** Medications with no mention of alcohol, but don't say   alcohol free.
    Tolu-Sed DM Cough Syrup (OTC, has 10% alcohol)
  * Sosufree Cough Syrup (OTC, alcohol free)
    Ryna-CX Liquid (CIV, alcohol free)
    Robitussin CF Liquid (OTC, has 4.75% alcohol)
    Tuss-Organidin Elixir (CIV, 16% alcohol)

Tussus SF Cough Syrup (CIV, 12% alcohol)
** Tricoden Liquid (OTC)
Tuss-Organidin DM Elixir (RX, 15% alcohol)
Pyrralan Expectorant DM (OTC, 6.5 alcohol)
Codimal DM Syrup (OTC, 9% alcohol)
Cerose DM Expectorant (OTC, 2.5% alcohol)
* Noratuss 11 Liquid (OTC, alcohol and narcotic free)
* Ryna C Liquid (CIV, alcohol free)
** Isochlor Liquid (RX)
* Ryna Liquid (OTC, alcohol free)
Trind Liquid (OTC, 5% alcohol)
** Covanamine Liquid (OTC)
S-T Decongestant Liquid (RX, 2.3% alcohol)
** Hycomine Syrup (CIII)
* Conar Suspension (OTC, alcohol free)
* Spantuss Suspension (RX, alcohol free)
* Nasahist Liquid (OTC, alcohol free)
* Trimedine Liquid (OTC, alcohol free)
Bay-Ornade Liquid (RX, 5% alcohol)
Tuss-Ornade Liquid (RX, 5% alcohol)
** Lanatuss Expectorant (OTC)
** Conex Expectorant (OTC)
Certro-Cirose Liquid (CIV, 1.5% alcohol)
Entuss Expectorant Tablets (CIII)
* Codiclear DH Syrup (alcohol free)
* Entuss Expectorant (alcohol free)

The use of alcohol can be very detrimental to hypoglycemics as it inhibits the release of glucose into the bloodstream from the liver.

Cough/Cold Preparations Without Alcohol (most contain sugar):

Anamine Syrup(OTC)
Chlorofed Liquid (OTC)
Deconamine Syrup (OTC)
Fedahist Syrup (OTC)
Ryna Liquid (OTC)
Triaminic Syrup (OTC)
Triaminic DM Liquid (OTC)
* Ryna C Liquid (CIV, sugar free)

Tussar DM Cough Syrup (OTC)
Fedahist Expectorant (OTC)
Kolephrin GG/DM Liquid (OTC)
Silexin Cough Syrup
* Sosufree Cough Mixture (OTC, narcotic and sugar free)
* Ryna CX Liquid (CIV, sugar free)
* Noratuss Liquid (OTC, sugar and narcotic free)
* Codiclear DH Syrup (CIII, sugar free)
* Entuss Expectorant (CII, sugar free)
Kolephrin NN Liquid (OTC)
* Tylenol (sugar free)

Caffeine causes the adrenal glands to stimulate the liver to release glucose into the bloodstream.

These Products contain sugar, or alcohol, or both:

Emprazil 30 mg.(RX)
Fendal 32.6 mg.(OTC)
Emagrin Forte 32.8 mg.(OTC)
Bowman Gold Tablets 16 mg.(OTC)
Salete-D Caps. 16 mg.(OTC)
Drinophen Caps. 15 mg.(OTC)
Efed 11 Caps. 125 mg.(OTC)
Phenetron Compound 30 mg.(OTC)
Dasikon Caps. 32 mg.(OTC)
Coriforte Caps. 30 mg.(RX)
Dilone 30 mg.(OTC)
Medache 32 mg.(OTC)
Triaminicin 30 mg.(OTC)
Dristan Caps. & Tablets 16.2 mg.(OTC)
Sinapils Tablets 32.5 mg.(OTC)
Kolephrine 65 mg.(OTC)
Duradyne Forte 30 mg.(OTC)
Cenaid 10 mg.(OTC)
Sinexin 32.5 mg.(OTC)
Korigesic 30 mg.(RX)
Valihist 45 mg.(OTC)
Histosal 30 mg.(OTC)
Coryban-D 30 mg.(OTC)

Super-Decon 32 mg.(OTC)
Citra 30 mg.(OTC)
Citra Forte 30 mg.(CIII)
Hycomine Compound 30 mg.(CIII)
Omnicol 10 mg.(RX)
Tussirex @ Codeine Liquid 25 mg.(CIV)
Kolephrine/DM Capsules 65 mg.(OTC)
Vivarin (OTC)

Be sure to read all labels of over the counter medicines or ask your Pharmacist for side effects and if the medication your doctor prescribed contain sugar.

Cooking Utensils

Recommended:
Stainless Steel
Glass
Ceramic
Cast Iron
Wooden Utensils
Stainless Utensils

Not recommended:
Aluminum
Teflon Coated Products

All aluminum should be avoided. This includes cooking with aluminum foil, aluminum cans, even products consumed which contain aluminum ingredients should be avoided, including deodorants and antiperspirants. Aluminum has been linked to Alzheimer's Disease. People who consume soft drinks should purchase them in glass or plastic bottles.

Conversion Tables

Sweeteners:

Equal Tablets — 25 tablets = 1 cup sugar
    2 tablets = 1 calorie
Fruit Sweeteners — 1/2 cup = 1 cup sugar
    1 Tablespoon = 57 calories = 15 grams Carbohydrates
Rice Syrup — 1/2 cup = 1 cup sugar
    1 Tablespoon = 86 calories = 22 grams Carbohydrates
Barley Malt — 1/4 cup = 1 cup sugar

Oils:

Shortening or butter		Vegetable Oils		Olive Oils
1 Tablespoon	=	1 TBSP.	or	1 TBSP.
2 Tablespoons	=	1 1/2 TBSP.	or	1 1/2 TBSP.
4 Tablespoons	=	3 TBSP.	or	2 1/2 TBSP.
1/3 cup	=	4 TBSP.	or	3 1/2 TBSP.
1/2 cup	=	6 TBSP.	or	5 1/2 TBSP.
1 cup	=	3/4 cup	or	1/2 cup

Table of Measures:

1 tsp.	=			4 milligrams
1 Tbsp.	=			15 milligrams
1/4 cup	=	4 Tbsp.	=	60 milligrams
1/3 cup	=	5 1/3 Tbsp.	=	79.95 milligrams
1/2 cup	=	8 Tbsp.	=	120 milligrams
2/3 cup	=	10.7 Tbsp.	=	160.5 milligrams
3/4 cup	=	12 Tbsp.	=	180 milligrams
1 cup	=	16 Tbsp.	=	240 milligrams
1 oz.	=			28.35 grams
1 lb.	=			454 grams

CHAPTER 7

Diet Plans with Daily Menus

With Dr. Manso's approval, I have developed the following diet plans for both myself and the clients that come in for counseling. The following are diet plans of approximately 1500, 1200, and 1000 calories. If these help you as much as they have helped others, I know you will have embarked on the road back to better health. All plans include a complete breakdown of total calories, complex carbohydrates, proteins, and fats.

Diet Plan #1 — 1500 Calories

Upon Rising:

Juice of 1 lemon with 8 oz. pure water

Calories — 17
Protein — 1
Fat — 0
Comp.Carb. — 5

Breakfast:

1 cup Oatmeal (cooked)
2 Slice Ezekiel Bread-Topped
1/2 tsp. no sugar jam per slice
1 cup Herb tea

Calories — 321
Comp.Carb. — 55
Protein — 16
Fat — 4

Mid-Morning:
1 Fresh Fruit (Peach)
2 tsp. Sesame Seeds

Calories — 86
Comp.Carb. — 19
Protein — 2
Fat — 4

Lunch:
Green Salad (see recipe)
2 cups Vegetable Soup

Calories — 170
Comp.Carb — 35
Protein — 4
Fat — 2

Mid-Afternoon:
1—8.45 oz. Westsoy Lite
Natural Soy Drink
Fruit Salad (1/4 Apple,
    1/2 Orange,
    1/4 cup Crushed Pineapple)

Calories — 255
Comp.Carb. — 49
Protein — 11
Fat — 2

Dinner:
4 oz. Baked Snapper
1 cup Steamed Broccoli
1/2 cup Steamed Carrots
1/2 Baked Sweet Potato

Calories — 208
Comp.Carb. — 30
Protein — 25
Fat — 2

After Dinner:
1 cup Fresh Strawberries

Calories — 45
Comp.Carb. — 10
Protein — 1
Fat — 1

Bedtime:
1 cup Hot Carob Drink (see recipe)
1 slice Ezekiel Bread topped
with 1 tbs peanut butter

Calories — 347
Comp.Carb. — 56
Protein — 9
Fat — 1

Total Calories: 1449
Total Complex Carbohydrates: 259 gms.
Total Protein: 58 gms.
Total Fat: 25 gms.

Approximate Breakdown, 1500 calorie diet:
Fat: 10-15% = 150-225 calories = 17-25 gms.
Protein: 15-20% = 225-300 calories = 56-75 gms.
Complex Carbohydrates: 60-65% = 900-975 calories = 225-244 gms.

Diet Plan #2 — 1500 Calories

Upon Rising:

4 oz. Vegetarian Protein Drink

Calories — 56
Comp.Carb. — 8
Protein — 4
Fat — 0

Breakfast:

4 Buckwheat Pancakes
2 Tbsp. Rice Syrup

Calories — 408
Comp.Carb. — 76
Protein — 18
Fat — 8

Mid-Morning:

1/2 Grapefruit
4 oz. Vegetarian Protein Drink

Calories — 75
Comp.Carb. — 19
Protein — 5
Fat — 0

Lunch:

1/2 cup Pasta Salad (see recipe)
2 cups Garden Pea Soup

Calories — 326
Comp.Carb. — 48
Protein — 23
Fat — 8

Mid-Afternoon:

4 oz. Vegetarian Protein Drink
2 cups Popcorn

Calories — 164
Comp.Carb. — 29
Protein — 8
Fat — 0

Dinner:

1 cup Cucumber Soup (see recipe)
1 serving Fish with Tahini sauce

Calories — 335
Comp.Carb. — 26

(4 oz.) 1/2 Baked Potato w/skin	Protein — 29
	Fat — 7

After Dinner:
    1/2 small Cantaloupe
    1/2 cup Nonfat Yogurt(plain)

Calories — 149
Comp.Carb. — 30
Protein — 8
Fat — 0

Bedtime:
    4 oz. Vegetarian Protein Drink

Calories — 56
Comp.Carb. — 8
Protein — 4
Fat — 0

Total Calories: 1569
Total Complex Carbohydrates: 244 gms.
Total Protein: 99 gms.
Total Fat: 23 gms.

Approximate Breakdown: 1500 calorie diet
Fat: 10-15% = 150-225 calories = 17-25 gms.
Protein: 25-30% = 375-450 calories = 94-113 gms.
Comp. Carbohydrates: 60-65% = 900-975 calories= 225-244 gms.

Diet Plan #3 — 1500 Calories

Upon Rising:
    Juice of 1 Lemon in 8 oz. pure water

Calories — 17
Comp.Carb. — 5
Protein — 1
Fat — 0

Breakfast:
    2 eggs Poached
    2 slices Homemade or Ezekiel Bread
      each topped with 1/2 tsp.
      no sugar jam
    1 cup Herbal Tea

Calories — 308
Comp.Carb. — 34
Protein — 18
Fat — 14

Mid-Morning:

8 oz. Banana Soy Slush (see recipe)
1 oz. Health Valley Herb Stone (from health food store)
Wheat Crackers topped with 1 tsp. no-sugar jam

Calories — 290
Comp.Carb. — 51
Protein — 7
Fat — 8

Lunch:

1 cup Whole Wheat Pasta with
1 Tbsp. Pesto Pasta Dressing (see recipe)
1 serving Green & Raw Vegetable Salad (see recipe)

Calories — 215
Comp.Carb. — 52
Protein — 5
Fat — 2

Mid-Afternoon:

1 cup chopped raw broccoli
1 raw carrot-chopped

Calories — 77
Comp.Carb. — 16
Protein — 6
Fat — 0

Dinner:

1 cup DeBoles Jerusalem Artichoke Spaghetti topped with 4 oz. Ragu Homestyle Spaghetti Sauce (no-sugar-added brand)
1 serving Green & Raw Vegetable Salad (see recipe)

Calories — 323
Comp.Carb.- 70
Protein — 9
Fat — 3.5

After Dinner:

1 cup Fresh Strawberries

Calories — 45
Comp.Carb. — 10
Protein — 1
Fat — 1

Bedtime:

8 oz. Banana Soy Slush (see recipe)

Calories — 153
Comp.Carb. — 30
Protein — 5
Fat — 2

Total Calories: 1428
Total Complex Carbohydrates: 268 gms.
Total Protein: 52 gms.
Total Fat: 30 gms.

Approximate Breakdown: 1500 calorie diet
Fat: 10-20% = 150-300 calories = 17-33 gms.
Protein: 15-20% = 225-300 calories = 56-75 gms.
Comp. Carbohydrates: 60-65% = 900-975 calories = 225-244 gms.

Diet Plan #4 — 1200 Calories

Upon Rising:

Juice of 1 Lemon in 8 oz. pure water

Calories — 17
Comp.Carb. — 5
Protein — 1
Fat — 0

Breakfast:

1/2 cup Oatmeal (cooked)
1 slice Ezekiel Bread-topped with
   1/2 tsp. no sugar jam
1 cup Herbal Tea

Calories — 152
Comp.Carb. — 26
Protein — 8
Fat — 1

Mid-Morning:

1 Fresh Orange
1 Tbs. pumpkin seeds

Calories — 134
Comp.Carb. — 16
Protein — 4
Fat — 7

Lunch:

Green Vegetable Salad (see recipe)
1 cup Vegetable Soup (see recipe)

Calories — 134
Comp.Carb. — 28
Protein — 2
Fat — 1

Mid-Afternoon:

1-8.45 oz. Westsoy Lite Natural
   Soy Drink
Fruit Salad (1/4 apple, 1/4 orange,
   1/4 cup crushed pineapple

Calories — 255
Comp.Carb. — 49
Protein — 11
Fat — 2

Dinner:

3 oz. Baked Snapper

Calories — 188

1/2 cup Steamed Broccoli	Comp.Carb. — 24
1/2 cup Steamed Carrots	Protein — 21
1/2 Baked Sweet Potato(medium)	Fat — 2

After Dinner:
1 cup Fresh Strawberries

Calories — 45
Comp.Carb. — 10
Protein — 1
Fat — 1

Bedtime:
1 cup Hot Carob Drink (see recipe)
1/2 slice Ezekiel Bread topped
   with 1 tsp. peanut butter

Calories — 324
Comp.Carb. — 61
Protein — 7
Fat — 6

Total Calories: 1249
Total Complex Carbohydrates: 219 gms.
Total Protein: 55 gms.
Total Fat: 20 gms.

Approximate Breakdown: 1200 calorie diet
Fat: 10-15% = 120-180 calories = 13-20 gms.
Protein: 22-25% = 240-300 calories = 60-75 gms.
Comp.Carbohydrates: 65-75% = 780-900 calories = 195-225 gms.

Diet Plan #5 — 1000 Calories

Upon Rising:
2 oz. Vegetarian Protein Drink

Calories — 28
Comp.Carb. — 5
Protein — 2
Fat — 0

Breakfast:
2 Buckwheat Pancakes Topped with
1 Tbsp. Rice Syrup
1 cup Herbal Tea

Calories — 204
Comp.Carb. — 38
Protein — 9
Fat — 4

Mid-Morning:

1/2 Grapefruit	Calories — 47
2 oz. Vegetarian Protein Drink	Comp.Carb. — 16
	Protein — 3
	Fat — 0

Lunch:

1/2 cup Pasta Salad (see recipe)	Calories — 86
served over bed of Romaine lettuce	Comp.Carb. — 6
	Protein — 7
	Fat — 6

Mid-Afternoon

3 oz. Vegetarian Protein Drink	Calories — 96
1 cup Popcorn	Comp.Carb. — 18
	Protein — 4
	Fat — 0

Dinner:

1 cup Cucumber Soup (see recipe)	Calories — 296
1 serving Fish with Tahini Sauce (3 oz)	Comp.Carb. — 25
(see recipe)	Protein — 23
1/2 Baked Potato with Skin	Fat — 6

After Dinner:

1/2 small Cantaloupe	Calories — 149
1/2 cup Non-Fat Yogurt (plain)	Comp.Carb. — 30
	Protein — 8
	Fat — 0

Bedtime:

4 oz. Vegetarian Protein Drink	Calories — 56
	Comp.Carb. — 8
	Protein — 4
	Fat — 0

Total Calories: 962
Total Complex Carbohydrates: 146 gms.
Total Protein: 60 gms.
Total Fat: 16 gms.

Approximate Breakdown: 1000 calorie diet
Fat: 10-15% = 100-150 calories = 11-17 gms.
Protein: 25-30% = 250-300 calories = 63-75 gms.
Comp.Carbohydrates: 60-65%= 600-650 calories= 150-163 gms.

Diet Plan # 6 — 1000 Calories

Upon Rising:
Juice of 1 Lemon in 8 oz. pure water

Calories — 17
Comp.Carb. — 5
Protein — 1
Fat — 0

Breakfast:
1 egg Poached
1 slice Homemade or Ezekiel Bread
1 cup Herbal Tea

Calories — 145
Comp.Carb. — 15
Protein — 9
Fat — 7

Mid-Morning:
4 oz. bowl of Health Valley 100%
Natural Minestrone Soup
    (from health food store)

Calories — 90
Comp.Carb. — 10
Protein — 3
Fat — 4

Lunch:
1 cup Whole Wheat Pasta with 1 Tbsp
Pesto Pasta Dressing (see recipe)
1/2 serving of Green Raw Vegetable Salad
    (see recipe)

Calories — 166
Comp.Carb. — 42
Protein — 5
Fat — 2

Mid-Afternoon:
1 Fresh Peach

Calories — 37
Comp.Carb. — 10
Protein — 1
Fat — 0

Dinner:

1 cup DeBoles Jerusalem Artichoke
Spaghetti topped with 4 oz.
Ragu Homestyle Spaghetti Sauce
   (no-sugar-added brand)
1 serving of Green & Raw Vegetable Salad
   (see recipe)

Calories — 274
Comp.Carb. — 60
Protein — 9
Fat — 3

After Dinner:

1 cup Fresh Strawberries

Calories — 45
Comp.Carb. — 10
Protein — 1
Fat — 0

Bedtime:

1 slice Cornbread
8 oz. Westsoy Natural Soy Drink

Calories — 265
Comp.Carb. — 34
Protein — 7
Fat — 6

Total Calories: 1039
Total Complex Carbohydrates: 186 gms.
Total Protein: 36 gms.
Total Fat: 22 gms.

Approximate Breakdown: 1000 calorie diet
Fat: 10-20% = 100-200 calories = 11-22 gms.
Protein: 15-20% = 150-200 calories = 37-50 gms.
Comp.Carbohydrates: 65-75% = 650-750 calories = 163-188 gms.

CHAPTER 8

AN INTRODUCTION TO HEALTH AND FITNESS

Carbohydrates, Proteins and Fats

Your body is your tool; it is important to know what it requires for energy and upkeep. Carbohydrates, fats, and proteins all provide energy for your body. We measure the energy value in food by calories; the more calories in a particular food, the more energy it will produce in your body, or the more fat will be created if your caloric intake exceeds what your body needs.

Carbohydrates: Supply the most efficient source of energy. They are converted to sugars and are stored in the muscles as glycogen and in the blood as glucose. Glycogen is the energy source that drives our muscles, while glucose is one of the substances in our blood that regulates our body functions. Because carbohydrates are swiftly converted to glycogen and glucose, they give us quick energy after eating them.

Protein: Builds and repairs tissues that are broken down during exercise. One gram of protein for every kilogram (2.2 lbs.) of body weight will meet one's daily needs. This translates into, for example, a 120 lbs. person needing approximately 55 grams of protein per day.

Fat: Fat stored in the body is an energy reserve to protect us from running out of calories. Fat also aids in various bio-chemical reactions in the body. While a small amount of fat is necessary for good health, too much fat is harmful.

Fat is very concentrated energy. As a rough comparison, fat provides about 2-3 times as many calories for a given weight as do complex carbohydrates and proteins.

Recommended:
**Complex Carbohydrates should make up 60-80% of your total calories.
**Protein should make up 10-20% of your total calories.
**Fat should make up 10-20% of your total calories.

Getting Fit and Staying Fit

What is fitness? Obviously fitness means different things to different people. Although a small percentage of my clients are underweight, I would have to say that the majority of them are overweight. It would be great if I could offer you the magic answer to this problem, but unfortunately, there isn't any.

As we all know, there are many different diets out on the market, and in reality none of these work. Fad diets in themselves convey the idea that this is a temporary situation, but there is no temporary solution to the problem of being overweight.

To understand the problem, we must first understand how our bodies work. Studies show that we are governed by a metabolic clock which is set at a certain weight. If we go on a diet for a short period of time, we will lose weight, but the problem is that we won't keep it off. Anyone can lose weight; keeping the weight off is the problem.

Let's assume your weight loss goal is fifteen pounds. After you have lost these unwanted pounds, you will feel really good about yourself. Your clothes fit better, you can bend over much easier and you now feel that the battle has been won. During the diet you deprived yourself of having lunch with your friends or resisted the urge to have that special dessert. Now that the weight is off, you feel that you can again indulge yourself in the simple pleasures of life.

Slowly but surely you begin to slip right back into those old eating habits that had caused you to be overweight in the first place. Before you realize it, those unwanted pounds begin to slip right back on. Only this time you will gain an additional five to ten extra pounds because your body doesn't know when you are going to go off the edge again and decide to starve yourself, so it is going to protect itself against the next famine. This is called self-preservation.

Discouraging, isn't it? How in the world do we achieve that weight loss, and more importantly, how do we keep off those unwanted pounds?

There is no magic pill. We must keep our intake of calories in balance with the amount of calories that we burn for energy. With an intake of just ten extra calories per day in excess of the amount your body burns off for energy, you will add an extra twenty pounds to your body in just one year. If you have been slowly gaining weight over the past ten years, it is unrealistic to expect to lose that excess weight in a short period of time, much less expect to keep it off. One's objective should be to quit gaining weight today and work on losing that excess weight tomorrow. If you have added an extra ten pounds to your body over the past several years, you may need to re-examine your caloric intake as well as your activity level.

There are no short cuts. At least half of the calories you have consumed must be burned off in some sort of exercise or activity. When you are placed on a 1000 calorie per day program, instead of your usual 2000 calories per day, it will take 3.5 days to lose one pound of fat, and 7 days to lose two pounds of fat. You will have to work off 3500 calories to lose one pound of fat. One should shoot for a weight loss of no more than two pounds per week. Losing weight at this rate is the safe way of losing. By allowing the metabolism to slowly adjust to the weight loss, your body will be losing mostly fat instead of muscle during this period. This is where the balance in your activity level is so important. Reaching your goal and maintaining that goal for at least a period of one year can mean the difference between success and failure. *Holding your weight within three to four pounds of your goal weight for at least one year should reset your metabolic clock.* You won't rush back so easily into that weight gain situation. Maintaining this new lifestyle for at least one year after your weight goal has been reached should set the pattern for a lifetime.

Many people will lose and gain hundreds of pounds over a lifetime. It is healthier to stay heavy rather than have constantly fluctuating weight. The battle of the bulge is truly a lifetime commitment.

Skipping meals or eating very little will not help you lose those extra pounds. Skipping or scrimping on your food intake will lower your basal metabolic rate (BMR). The BMR is the minimum energy required to sustain your body's vital functions at rest. When this is lowered, your body's caloric requirement is automatically reduced. This means that when you skip meals or scrimp on food, you are making it harder for yourself to lose that weight.

Whether we are hypoglycemic, diabetic, overweight, or underweight, good nutrition will benefit everyone. It is unfortunate that most of us have to have some problem before we realize that better nutritional habits have to be addressed. Proper nutrition can do wonders for us. Whether we need to lose weight, gain weight, or just feel healthier, it will happen.

How to Figure Your Caloric Needs

Step One:

Multiply your goal weight by one of these factors:

	Women	Men
Under age 45	10 calories	11 calories
Over age 45	9 calorie	10 calories

Example: A woman over 45 years old: 130 lbs.(goal weight) x 9 calories/lb. = 1170 calories.

The figure 1170 represents the calories needed for basal metabolism (energy required while at-rest).

Step Two:

Multiply the above figure of 1170 by one of the following factors to cover calorie needs for activity: 0.5 for moderate activity and 0.3 if you are sedentary.

Example: 1170 x 0.5 = 850 additional calories.

Add this 850 calories to the 1170 calories needed for basal metabolism: 1170 + 850 = 2020 calories. This makes a total of 2020 calories per day to maintain a weight of 130 pounds with moderate activity.

Step Three:

To lose one pound per week, you will need to consume 500 calories less per day. To lose two pounds per week, you will need to consume 1000 calories less per day.

Example: 2020 - 500 = 1520 calories; or 2020 - 1000 = 1020 calories.

To gain one pound per week, instead of subtracting, you will need to add 750 calories per day to your daily maintenance calorie total.

Example: 2020 + 750 = 2770 calories.

> You should never go below 1000 calories per day to lose weight.

How Many Calories Does Exercise Use?

Here is the formula to help determine how many calories you will use up from exercise: Multiply your body weight X the exercise conversion factor (from the chart below). Multiply this figure X the number of minutes you exercise.

Activity	Conversion Factor
Aerobic dancing	.076
Circuit weight training	.085
Cycling (leisure)	.054
Gardening	.044
Golfing	.038
Jogging	.062
Rowing (machine)	.046
Skiing (cross-country)	.065
Swimming (leisure)	.058
Tennis	.050
Walking (leisure)	.037
Walking (briskly, or up and down hills)	.055

For example, if you weigh 135 lbs. and you do a brisk walk for 45 minutes: 135 lbs X .055 = 7.425 X 45 minutes = 334 calories used.

Your goal should be to burn at least 500 calories per day through exercise. These calories don't have to be expended all at once. Alternate your activities to avoid boredom. Enjoy whatever exercise you are involved in!

Body Fat

How much fat should we have on our bodies? The following chart should help you to understand how much fat you should have on your body. Fat is your body's insulation for the internal organs, and helps protect you against injury and infection. Fat also protects your body's internal thermostat. Too much fat is not healthy for anyone. Few people can live up to the ideal body fat recommended, unless they happen to be an athlete. For this reason, I recommend that you strive for the "healthy" level of body fat, which is more realistic.

Too often our goals are not realistic and when we fail to achieve these goals, we tend to get very discouraged and often quit trying. Achieving and maintaining your ideal body weight and body fat should be a life-long commitment for all of us.

	% of Body Fat	
Weight Condition	**Women**	**Men**
Ideal:	18-22%	15-18%
Healthy:	20-25%	15-21%
Average:	18-34%	11-24%
Healthy Obese:	30%	25%
Unhealthy Obese:	31-60%	26-50%
Morbid Obesity:	above 60%	above 50%

Dieting without exercise will give you only a 50% result. Only when you combine both dieting and exercise do you achieve 100% results. An aerobic exercise program will be effective in burning the intermuscular fat, therefore promoting weight loss and also preventing you from losing muscle. You will also burn more calories when you exercise because your basal metabolic rate (BMR) is increased by approximately 10% with a regular aerobics program. This means that even while you are asleep you will burn more calories.

Initiating an aerobic exercise program three or four times per week along with exercises for toning and firming the muscles will give you excellent results. As we grow older, it is even more important that we exercise on a regular basis, not only for weight control, but for better overall health. Studies have proven that without exercise an individual will lose an estimated two pounds of muscle per year, which is replaced by fat. As the years go by, this can make a big difference in the contour of our bodies.

Getting older doesn't necessarily mean we have to accept a flabby body. The muscular system supports the skeletal system. As we grow older, it is more important than ever to have strong firm muscles for proper function.

It is no longer believed that one has to work till one drops to get results. In fact, if you are exhausted or starved after your workout, you have worked too hard. Working at the right intensity will burn the intermuscular fat as your primary fuel source, while working at too high an intensity burns the glycogen, which is the stored energy within the muscle. This is why you will feel muscular weakness, or fatigue and even hunger after too intense a workout. Overworking will in fact defeat your purpose.

For the hypoglycemic or diabetic, there is no other choice to make. Whichever program works for you, make it one you can enjoy. We can all find time for the important things in our lives. It all depends on how badly we want to feel good. Remember, no one has the time to exercise— we all have to make the time!

Spot reducing doesn't work. You can't turn fat into muscle. Fat cells are composed of oily lipids (fats). Muscle cells are mostly water and protein. They are genetically and structurally different tissue and can't interchange. If you expend more calories than you take in, then your body can be forced to call on its energy stores, "its fat cells," to make up the balance. This usage isn't specified to a certain area of the body; it is overall. The fat lying on top of the muscle doesn't belong to that particular muscle; it belongs to the entire body.

In women, fat commonly is invested first on the thighs, hips, and lower torso, then to the upper body, particularly to the upper arms. On men the primary area where fat builds up is the mid-abdomen and all around the waist. When you are on a weight loss program, the deposits of fat are removed in the reverse order.

So how do you take off that UNWANTED FAT? One could simply diet, and if you really stayed with it, you would lose weight, but the body would appear flabby and that would be very discouraging. Unless an exercise program is included with your weight loss program, the results will not be 100% effective. You also lose less muscle tone if you are exercising while you are losing weight. To lose fat you must first mobilize the fatty acid from the fat cell, and then utilize it! This means "Aerobic Exercise!" The medium-intense, long lasting exertion of large muscle groups is what metabolizes (burns up) fat!

The best way to take fat off those hips, stomachs, or arms is through total-analysis aerobic exercise combined with a well-balanced diet. You need no magic pills—just common sense and hard work.

Starting an Exercise Program

Before initiating any exercise program, it is wise to consult with your physician, especially if you are on any type of medication or have any heart problems, diabetes, or high blood pressure. If you are over thirty-five, you should have a stress electrocardiogram before beginning your program. The main thing to remember is not to overdo. You know your limitations better than anyone else, and you will want to work within those limitations.

I taught public classes for several years and realized that it is extremely difficult for one instructor to do justice to a large class. It is hard to make anyone understand that they need to pace themselves in a workout. For the most part, people don't realize that they are overworking until it is too late. In a class, the energy is flowing, the music is loud, and you see the person next to you really working hard, so it is almost impossible not to be intimidated by this much energy. It is only when your body cools down, that you realize that you have worked too hard.

Very few people are able to go into a high impact aerobic class and remain injury free. In time, I believe the exercise industry will rule out all high impact aerobic classes, as they have ruled out so many of the unsafe exercises we used to do in the beginning. For anyone over thirty, the high impact workout is most unwise. I prefer to go with the low impact, or the non-impact aerobic workouts. In the long run, it is much safer and has been proven to be even more effective in weight reduction programs.

When I first started exercising, many years ago, we worked as hard as possible because we believed we would not achieve any results. Thank heavens the exercise industry has changed its attitudes about fitness. I can remember the morning after my first class. I felt as if I had been run over by a truck. I could hardly turn over in bed the next morning without feeling that I was going to die. I had obviously overworked, for it took me a week to get over the soreness. A good rule to remember is that if you are still sore 48 hours after your workout, you have overworked. I am not at all surprised at the dropout rate for the beginning exerciser when I remember my first workout. I soon decided that if I would ever get over these first few weeks, I would never stop exercising because I never wanted to go through that pain again. Let's face it, not many of us enjoy doing this to our bodies. As a professional instructor I always try to pace the beginner so you won't have to go through the pain I went through on my first experience with an exercise class.

So often the fitness industry is designed for the fit individual. The exercise classes or spas attract the fit and are often considered more of a place for social gatherings, which makes the overweight/overfat client very uncomfortable. As a personal trainer, I have the opportunity to work not only with the obese, but also with the elderly and often geriatric patient. Working with a client on a one to one basis gives me the opportunity to not only develop a personal relationship with that individual, but to really see the results that my program can offer.

For whatever the reason a person doesn't feel that he/she can or wants to go into a class atmosphere, a personal trainer can offer so much more, as far as quality of the workout, privacy, and individualized attention that can't be offered in a large class.

I don't advise anyone to exercise on a full stomach, but as a hypoglycemic, you can't go very long without eating. The food is your energy, so it is important that you eat a small amount of protein along with some complex carbohydrates an hour or so before you start any exercise routine.

One of the things you need to know about aerobic exercise is what is referred to as the heart *Target Rate*. To be totally effective, your exercises should increase the rate that your heart beats up to a given percentage of its maximum capacity.

For example, your resting heart rate before you begin the exercise program might be 72 beats per minute, and your maximum heart rate might be 175 beats per minute. The object of programmed aerobic exercise is not to work your heart at its maximum capacity, but at a certain pecentage of its capacity that is correct for you as a beginner.

Let's say, for example, that it is determined that your exercise program should enable you to sustain a heart rate at 60% of maximum, or 105 beats per minute. 105 beats per minute is your *Target Rate*, and this rate of 105 beats per minute is what your exercise program will be designed to sustain over a certain number of minutes.

The chart below shows some typical Target Rates for persons of different ages.

Age	Moderate Intensity - 60%	Intermediate Intensity- 70%	Athletic Range -80%
15	123	143	164
25	117	136	156
35	111	129	148
45	105	122	140
55	99	115	132
65	93	108	124

These figures are based on an average resting heart rate of 80 beats per minute for women and 72 beats per minute for men.

In order to figure out what your Target Zone will be, you will need to know your resting heart rate. Early in the morning is the best time to take your resting pulse. Before getting out of bed in the morning or before moving around much, find your pulse by placing your fingertips against your wrists to find your radial pulse, or against the side of the neck to find your carotid pulse. Do not use your thumb because the thumb has a pulse of its own and you won't get an accurate reading. I suggest you use the index finger and the middle finger, placed lightly against the pulse and count each heartbeat for 60 seconds. You may want to add the figure for three days in a row and then divide the total by three. This should give you a pretty good average of what your resting heart rate is.

As a beginner a good place to start is an intensity of 60-65%. Here is a way to determine your Target Rate:

1) Maximum heart rate (MHR) = 220 minus your age.

2) MHR minus your resting heart rate (RHR) x intensity %.

3) Add your RHR to the result of Step 2.

Example:

1) 220 minus your age of 44 years = MHR of 176.

2) 176 minus your RHR of 81 = 95 x 60% = 57.

3) 81 + 57 = 138.

For this example, the Target Rate is 138 beats per minute.

Using the above example, This 44-year-old woman should work at a target rate of 138 for at least four days per week in her aerobic program. While exercising, you will need to take your pulse. If you were to stop for a full 60 seconds or even for 15 seconds, your heart rate would slow down and you would not get an accurate reading. This is why it is recommended that you stop and count your pulse for 10 seconds and multiply that by 6. This will give an accurate heart rate without giving your heart a chance to slow down.

You will want to check your pulse during your workout. DO NOT OVERWORK. After you become accustomed to the aerobic workout, you will not need to check your heart rate so often, but you want to be careful at first. Only during the aerobic workout will it be necessary to check your heart rate so closely. During the other workouts, check it periodically to make sure you are not overworking.

It would be wise for anyone with any heart problems or over forty years of age to check with their physician and have a stress electrocardiogram before starting any exercise program. If you have heart problems, you will need to monitor your heart rate closely and not exceed the maximum recommended rate.

If you are a beginner, the aerobic part of the workout should be at least twenty minutes, then as your stamina improves you can increase the workout to thirty minutes and, finally, to forty-five minutes.

Injuries and Exercise Safety

If you will be working out on a daily basis, one good way is to do aerobics and toning (stretches) on alternate days. If weights are used, they should be used only every other day. This will allow the connective tissue to repair itself and recuperate from the demand you have placed upon your muscles. Stretches can be done on a daily basis, but remember that the body should be allowed to warm up first, even for stretches. It is important to take at least two minutes or so before your workout for marching in place, breathing deeply, and moving your arms. This will elevate the body's temperature and warm up these muscles so as not to cause injury. The aerobic part of the workout should be done at least three, and preferably four, days per week, especially if you need to lose weight.

Studies show that it will take at least one year to get into shape. After you have achieved your goal, exercising at least three times per week will keep you in shape.

Unfortunately, fitness cannot be stored without exercising. You will need to continue with your exercise program in order to have the benefit of a firm, healthy body. The sad fact is that within just three weeks after discontinuing your exercise program you will begin to lose the muscle tone that took a year to build up.

For the beginner the aerobic part of the workout should be at least 20 minutes. Then, as your stamina improves, you can increase your workout to 30 minutes. Depending on your condition and how much weight you have to lose, I usually recommend a 45-minute aerobic program.

Here are some safety tips: never use your weights during the warmup or cooldown segments of your workout; and never use ankle weights during the aerobics section. These practices can result in excessive impact shock on the musculoskeletal system. When weights are used, you should be careful not to work at too high an intensity-such as jumping jacks, high kicks and lunges, or high-level jogging. An aerobic dance class averages five times normal body weight for each step. It is no surprise that in a high-impact jumping and hard jogging class, injuries can and often do occur. Studies have shown that 60-83% of injuries occur below the knee.

It has also been proven through research that once a certain level of fitness has been achieved, continued large improvements cannot be expected. Therefore, the exerciser who seeks to increase intensity with high impact movements will often experience injury rather than improvement.

Tips on Fitness

Aerobic exercises are important to burn fat & maintain cardiorespiratory fitness, but equally important is your floor work (toning). If any of my private students haven't exercised in a long time, I will never start them with an aerobic workout. The first three to six weeks will be devoted to floor work. It is important to strengthen your muscles and gain flexibility before we go into any aerobic program. Stronger and more flexible muscles are the biggest factors in injury prevention.

Indications are that people tend to stick with programs that involve lower intensity and longer duration. If your exercise program is painful and unpleasant or if you are so washed out that you can't go about your daily work load after your exercise program, you won't stick with it very long. We use this as an excuse because, too often, exercise is not at the top of our list anyway.

Approaching any changes in our regular habits isn't easy. Always remember to start slowly and work at your own pace with any of the exercises recommended in this book.

After your weight goal has been reached, I recommend you go from a four day a week workout, to a three day a week workout and continue with the 45-minute aerobic program. Working within your limitations and gradually pushing harder as your stamina improves give excellent results. I recommend that you discuss your exercise program with a certified professional instructor before getting started, so as to achieve the desired results.

Exercise stabilizes your blood sugar. This is one of the reasons you have so much energy after starting a regular exercise program. You will find your energy level will be higher throughout the day. Exercise changes your whole metabolism and will better enable you to control your blood sugar.

Exercise can do wonders for your total health. Not only will you look better, you will also feel better. There is no better way to relieve depression or fatigue than exercise. Whichever exercise program you choose, exercise is a must if you are to achieve a better and healthier lifestyle.

CHAPTER 9

THE EXERCISES

EXERCISES FOR RELAXATION AND FLEXIBILITY

1.
Stand tall, feet shoulder-width apart, knees relaxed, pelvis in, abdomen tight. Deeply inhale as you bring your arms up above your head, clasping hands together as you stretch up as high as you can. Keep your head straight forward, do not let head fall back. Stretch arms up high, feel that stretch throughout your entire body. As you slowly exhale through your mouth, release your arms and bring them down by your side. Repeat stretch three (3) times.

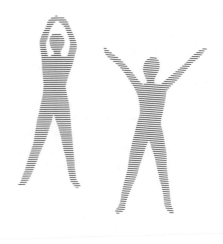

2.
Stand tall, feet shoulder-width apart, knees relaxed, pelvis in, abdomen tight, neck relaxed. Slowly roll shoulders back in large circular motion. Repeat roll three (3) times, then roll shoulders forward in the same manner three (3) times. Breathe deeply and slowly.

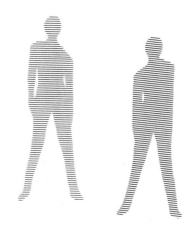

3a.
Stand tall, feet shoulder-width apart, knees relaxed, pelvis in, abdomen tight. Move arms and legs as in a fast walk. Continue marching in place for at least three (3) minutes. Relax.
NOTE: This exercise is important to warm the body temperature before you start your stretching exercises.

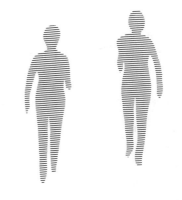

3b.
Stand tall, feet shoulder-width apart, knees relaxed, pelvis in, abdomen tight. Deeply inhale as you bring your arms above your head, clasping hands together as you stretch up as high as you can. Keep you head straight forward, do not let head fall back. Stretch arms up high, feel that stretch throughout your entire body. As you slowly exhale through your mouth, release your arms and bring them down by your side. Relax.

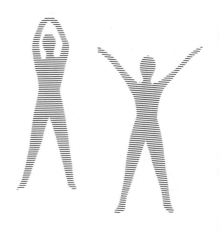

4.

Stand tall, feet shoulder-width apart, knees relaxed, pelvis in, abdomen tight. Gently hold your right elbow with your left hand, gently pull arm to the opposite shoulder while you slightly bend your right knee, relax your body as you enjoy this stretch. Hold stretch for thirty (30) seconds, repeat for other side. Breathe normally.

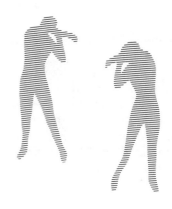

5.

Stand tall, feet shoulder-width apart, knees relaxed, pelvis in, abdomen tight. Hold on to your right wrist with your left hand as you bring your arm and elbow behind your head. Gently stretch arm back and to the side. Hold stretch for thirty (30) seconds. Relax. Repeat for other side. Feel stretch through triceps and upper back. Breathe normally.

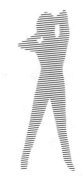

6.

Stand tall, feet shoulder-width apart, knees relaxed, pelvis in, abdomen tight. Interlace your fingers out in front of your body, shoulder level, palms turned outward. Deeply inhale and then slowly exhale, stretch arms outward from your body as far as you can. Hold the stretch for thirty (30) seconds. Relax. Feel the stretch through your shoulders, middle of upper back, arms, hands and wrists.

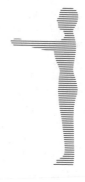

7.

Stand tall, feet shoulder-width
apart, knees relaxed, pelvis in,
abdomen tight. Bring right arm
over your head, gently pull head
down toward right shoulder, relax
head completely. Hold stretch for
thirty (30) seconds. Relax.
Repeat stretch for other side.
Breathe normally.

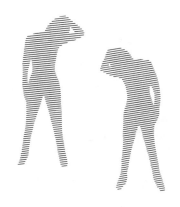

8.

Stand tall, feet shoulder-width
apart, knees relaxed, pelvis in,
abdomen tight. Slowly drop head
down, chin into chest. Bring both
hands behind your neck, letting
the weight of your arms gently pull
head down. Hold stretch for thirty
(30) seconds. Feel the stretch
down the back of the neck and upper
spine. Breathe normally.

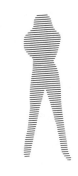

9.

Stand tall, feet shoulder-width apart,
knees relaxed, pelvis in, abdomen tight.
Slowly drop head down, chin into chest,
continue rolling your spine forward and
down one vertebra at a time, relax body
supporting your body with hands on
your legs. Hold position for thirty (30)
seconds, then slowly reverse the spinal
roll, rolling body slowly upward, one
vertebra at a time. Feel stretch
throughout the spine, helps to
elongate the back. Breathe normally.

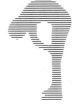

10.

Stand tall, feet wide apart, knees
relaxed, pelvis in, abdomen tight.
Deeply inhale as you lift both your
arms over your head, slowly exhale
through your mouth as you bring your
left arm over your head as far as
possible, as you slowly bend your
body to the right. Do not bend
elbow, just reach out to the side,
arm across your head. Place your
right hand against your right knee
to support your lower back. Hold
stretch for thirty (30) seconds.
Slowly return body to upright
position, repeat stretch for other
side. Feel stretch around waist
and down sides. Breathe slowly
while holding stretch.

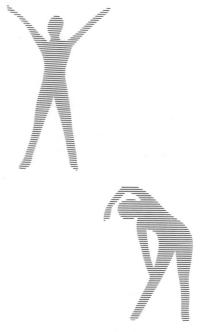

You may continue with the exercise I have outlined for the ankles,
calves, and quadriceps, then on to the exercises for the lower back. If you
have a weak lower back you will find these exercises I have outlined a
great relief. Do these stretching exercises every day before initiating any
workout or just in order to help you to relax. Within a matter of a few
weeks you will see a noticeable improvement in you flexibility.

EXERCISES FOR THE ANKLES, CALVES AND QUADRICEPS

1.

Sit on mat, with legs stretched out, feet flexed,
abdomen tight. Deeply inhale and then slowly
exhale, as you reach out to hold the balls of
the feet, keeping body and chin in a neutral
position. Do not hold head upward or down-
ward. Hold stretch for thirty (30) seconds. If you
are not very flexible, you may want to use a
towel around the bottom of your feet to help
with this stretch.

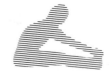

2.

Lie on your left side, resting
your head in the palm of your
hand, abdomen tight, body relaxed.
Bring your right foot back into
your body toward your right buttock.
Place right hand around right ankle,
deeply inhale and then slowly
exhale, as you gently pull your
right heel toward the right buttock,
keeping legs slightly apart. Hold
easy stretch for thirty (30) seconds.
Relax, repeat for other side.

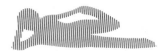

3.

Lying on mat, arms resting by your
sides, head held straight and
relaxed on mat. Cross your right
leg over, resting foot on top of
your left thigh. Flex your left
foot. Deeply inhale and then slowly
exhale as you bring your left leg
into your body. Hold stretch for
thirty (30) seconds, breathing
normally. Repeat for other leg.

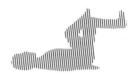

NOTE: A word of caution when getting up from a lying position. Always bring body into a fetal position, using elbows to support your upper body weight, push your body upward from the elbow onto your hands. Use your hands to support your body weight as you push your body into an upward position from your side.

EXERCISES FOR THE LOWER BACK

1.

Lay on mat or blanket. Lying
on your back, bring right knee
into body, foot flexed. Place
hands in back of leg just below
knee. Deeply inhale and then
slowly exhale as you pull leg
tighter into body. Hold stretch
for thirty (30) seconds, relax.
Repeat same stretch for other leg.
Never bring both legs into body at
the same time. This puts too much
stress on the lower back. Always
hold knee into body by placing hands
in back of leg, just below the knee.
This protects the delicate ligaments
and cartilage of the knee.

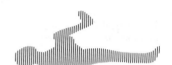

2.

Laying on your back, body relaxed,
bring right foot into body, with
left hand hold onto right ankle,
place right hand in back of right
knee. Deeply inhale and then slowly
exhale as you bring leg tighter into
body, holding firmly to foot and back
of leg. Hold stretch for thirty (30)
seconds, relax. Repeat the same
stretch for the other leg.

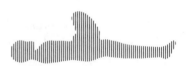

3.

Lying on your back, body relaxed,
bring both knees into chest, (one
at a time) slowly straighten legs
all the way up, feet flexed.
Place hands behind knees. Deeply
inhale and then slowly exhale as
you lift upper body slightly off
mat, bringing your head to your
knees while gently pulling back
on legs till you feel your
buttocks slightly lifting off
floor. Hold stretch for fifteen
(15) seconds. Relax. Repeat
two (2) times.

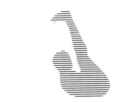

4.

Lying on your back, body relaxed,
bring both knees into chest, (one
leg at a time) feet flexed. Place
hands behind legs, just below knees.
Inhale deeply and then slowly exhale
as you tighten hold around legs,
till you feel buttocks slightly
lifting off floor. Hold stretch
for thirty (30) seconds. Relax.

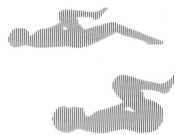

5a.

Lying on your back, body relaxed,
bring knees up, (one at a time)
keeping feet flat on the floor.
Extend arms over your head, resting
on floor. Bring your right leg
over the left leg, inhale deeply
and then slowly exhale, let your
legs fall slowly all the way over
to the left side. Hold stretch in
this position, and relax for thirty
(30) seconds, breathing normally.

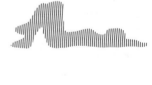

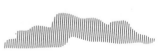

5b.

From position of Exercise 5A,
slowly bring both legs to the center
position still crossed, deeply inhale
and then slowly exhale as you let
your legs fall slowly all the way
over to the right side. Hold stretch
in this position, and relax for
thirty (30) seconds. Breathe
normally. Repeat stretch A and B
for other side, crossing left leg
over right leg. Excellent stretch
for the lower back and side of the
hip area.

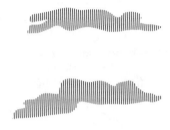

6a.

Lying on your back, body relaxed.
Bring knees into chest, (one at a
time) lying with head relaxed,
arms stretched out, knees together,
slowly rock legs from side to side.
Continue rocking motion for thirty
(30) seconds. Relax. Breathe
normally.

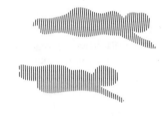

6b.

Lying on your back, body relaxed.
Bring knees into chest (one at a
time), feet flexed. Place hands
behind legs just below knees.
Inhale deeply and then slowly
exhale as you tighten hold around
legs, till you feel buttocks
slightly lifting off floor.
Hold stretch for thirty (30)
seconds. Relax.

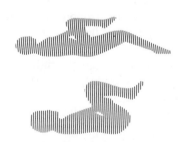

7.

Turn over onto your stomach, place
hands even with chest, legs stretched
out. Inhale deep then slowly exhale
as you slowly lift upper body,
keeping hips down, chin up. Hold
stretch for fifteen (15) seconds.
Repeat stretch one (1) time. Relax.

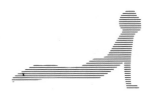

8.

Come up to hand and knees position.
Inhale deep as you round back as
high as you can, making waist as
small as you can, abdomen tight.
Slowly exhale as you stretch body
forward with chest flat on floor.
Relax, hold stretch for thirty (30)
seconds, breathe slowly.

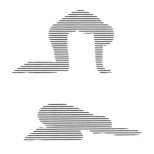

9.

From position in Exercise 8,
slowly roll body into upward position,
sitting back on your haunches with
toes curled under. Gently rock back
and forth with hands flat on floor
in front of you for support.
Breathe slowly, continue rocking
motion for thirty (30) seconds,
breathing normally. Relax.

10.

From position of Exercise 9, slowly
rock body back till feet are flat
on floor, body in squatting position.
Place hands on knees. Inhale
deeply then exhale slowly as you
push body upward with your hands,
letting your legs feel the weight
of your body as you lift upward one
vertebra at a time. Inhale deeply
as you bring your arms over your
head, slowly exhale as you bring
your arms down by your side.

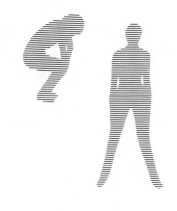

11.

Standing, bring your legs wide apart,
knees relaxed. Bring your left arm
down and over to grab your right
ankle. Extend your right arm upward
as your slightly turn your body and
your head slightly upward. Hold
stretch for thirty (30) seconds,
breathing normally. Repeat stretch
for other side.

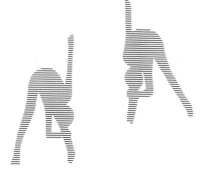

12.

Stand tall, feet shoulder-width
apart, knees relaxed, pelvis in,
abdomen tight. Inhale deeply as
you bring your arms up over your
head. Slowly exhale through your
mouth as you bring you arms back
down by your side. Relax.

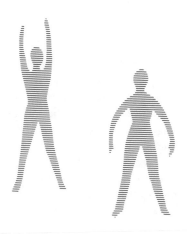

You may stop here or continue with the twenty (20) minute low level aerobic workout or work on alternate days with the exercises I have outlined to strengthen, tone and firm your muscles.

WEIGHTS

For the beginner I never recommend weights. It is important to strengthen the muscles before we can build. Only after you can do the routine with ease, do you add the free weights or the wrist weights. Start slow and work up. You want to work the muscles to the point of fatigue, not to the point of pain. If you don't feel the fatigue, you are not working hard enough. Remember to keep the fist closed and to work the arm tight. When you are using weights, remember the number of repetitions is more important than the amount of weight used.

If you are a woman, don't feel that you cannot work with weights because you will build heavy muscles like a man. In order to do that you would have to be taking special steroids, and use very heavy weights. What I suggest are light weights and more repetitions. This will help you to strengthen, tone and firm your muscles without fear of building large muscle bulk. Starting with one pound weights and working up to two and a half or three pound weights should give you the results you want without putting your body into too much stress. You will want to work with weights every other day. Keep in mind to work the arms as tight as you can, and resist as much as you can, but never hyper-extend the elbows. This is where you will see the results. If the muscles begin to burn or feel uncomfortable during any part of the exercises, you need to stop for a moment and relax, then pick it up again.

As your muscles become conditioned to the exercises, you will find you will be able to do more and work harder. Remember, you have to work up, so start slow, and don't give up.

Throughout the exercise, keep reminding yourself to stand tall with your abdominal muscles held in tight, and to keep the pelvis pulled in (do not push buttocks out). Concentrate on good posture. At all times your knees need to be relaxed, NEVER locked.

EXERCISES FOR THE BICEPS

1.

Stand tall, knees relaxed, feet shoulder-width apart, pelvis in, abdomen tight. Bring arms out to the side, shoulder level. Make a fist, now bend at the elbows and bring your fist in to touch your upper shoulders. Continue working arms in an in-out motion. Repeat ten (10) counts, work up to twenty-five (25). Inhale as you bring arms out, exhale as you bring arms in.

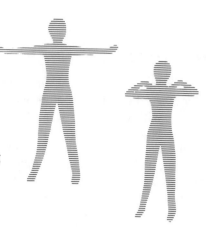

2.

Stand tall, knees relaxed, feet shoulder-width apart, pelvis in, abdomen tight. Bring arms out straight in front of your body, palms up, fists closed, shoulder level. Now bend at the elbows as you bring your fists in to touch your upper shoulders. Continue working arms in an in-out motion. Repeat ten (10) counts, work up to twenty-five (25). Inhale as you bring arms out, exhale as you bring arms in.

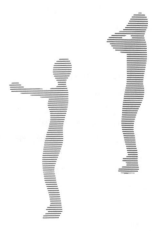

3.

Stand tall, knees relaxed, feet shoulder-width
apart, pelvis in, abdomen tight. Rest right
elbow on right hip, now bend arm at the
elbow as you bring fist up to touch your
right shoulder. Continue working arm in an
in-out motion. Repeat ten (10) counts, work
up to twenty-five (25) counts. Repeat for
other arm. Inhale as you bring arm out,
exhale as you bring arm in.

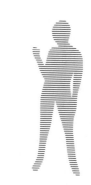

4.

Stand tall, knees relaxed, feet shoulder-width
apart, pelvis in, abdomen tight, fists closed.
Hold both arms out straight in front of your
body, palms up a little higher than shoulder
level. Now hold arms up as you resist as
tight as you can. Pretend you are trying to
hold up a very heavy weight. Hold tightness
for thirty (30) seconds, relax. Repeat five (5)
counts, work up to ten (10) counts. Inhale as
you bring arm up, exhale as you resist,
breathing normally as you hold.

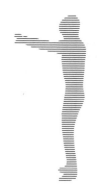

The Triceps:

5.

Stand tall, knees relaxed, feet
shoulder-width apart, pelvis in,
abdomen tight, fists closed. Bring right
arm up against right ear. Now bend arm
back at the elbow and bring fist to touch
back of upper shoulder. Continue
working arm in an in-up motion.
Repeat ten (10) counts, work up to
twenty (20). Repeat for left arm. Exhale
as you bring arm up, inhale as you
bring arm back.

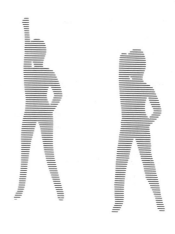

6.

Stand tall, knees relaxed, feet
shoulder-width apart, pelvis in,
abdomen tight, fists closed. Bring
both arms out straight in front of
your body, palms down, shoulder
level. Now bend arms at the elbows
as you bring your fists in to touch
your upper shoulders. Continue
working arms in an in-out motion.
Repeat ten (10) counts, work up to
twenty-five (25). Inhale as you bring
arms out, exhale as you bring arms in.

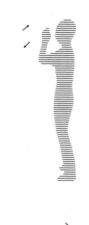

7.

Stand tall, knees relaxed, feet
shoulder-width apart, pelvis in,
abdomen tight. Clasp hands
together, lift both arms up above
your head. Now bend arms back at
the elbows as you bring clasped
hands to touch the back of the neck.
Continue working arms in an in-up
motion. Repeat ten (10) counts,
work up to twenty-five (25) counts.
Exhale as you bring arms up, inhale
as you bring arms in.

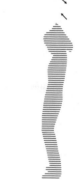

8.

Stand tall, knees relaxed, feet
shoulder-width apart, pelvis in,
abdomen tight. Assume same position
as in Exercise 7. As you bring arms up
bring them out in front of your body
at chest level, then back again so that
clasped hands touch the back of the
neck. Continue working in an
over-out motion. Repeat ten (10)
counts, work up to twenty-five (25)
counts. Exhale as you bring arms out
in front of your body, inhale as you
bring them back.

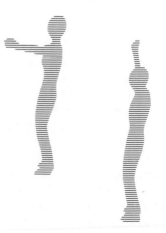

9.
Stand tall, knees relaxed, feet shoulder-width apart, pelvis in, abdomen tight, fists closed. Hold both arms out straight in front of your body, palms facing down, a little higher than shoulder level. Now hold arms out as you resist as tight as you can. Pretend you are trying to push down a heavy weight. Hold tightness for thirty (30) seconds, relax. Repeat five (5) counts, work up to ten (10) counts. Inhale as you bring arms up, exhale as you resist, breathe normally as you hold.

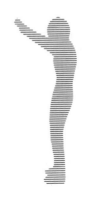

10.
Stand tall, knees relaxed, feet shoulder-width apart, pelvis in, abdomen tight, fist closed. Hold both arms out behind you, tight against your sides. Now push arms up from this position, resist as tight as you can, pretend you are trying to push arms up, holding up a heavy weight. Hold tightness for thirty (30) seconds, relax. Repeat five (5) counts, work up to ten (10) counts. Breathe normally as you hold.

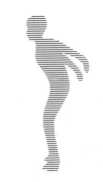

Pectoral Muscles:

11.
Stand tall, knees relaxed, feet shoulder-width apart, pelvis in, abdomen tight, fists closed. Bring arms straight out to the side, shoulder level. Bend arms at the elbow as you bring arms into chest. Arch chest slightly outward as you push arms out to the side again shoulder level. Continue working arms in an in-out motion. Repeat ten (10) counts, work up to twenty- five (25) counts. Inhale as you bring arms in, exhale as you bring arms out.

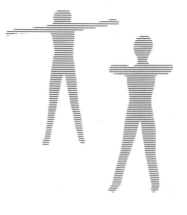

12.

Stand tall, knees relaxed, feet shoulder-width apart, pelvis in, abdomen tight, fists closed. Bring arms straight out in front of your body, shoulder level, arms together, elbows straight. Now push arms straight out to your sides, shoulder level. Continue pushing arms in an in-out motion. Repeat ten (10) counts. Inhale as you bring arms in, exhale as you push arms out.

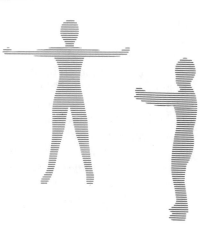

13.

Stand tall, knees relaxed, feet shoulder-width apart, abdomen tight, fists closed. Bring both arms out straight in front of your body at chest level. Bring arms in-out in a boxing type motion, relax and let your body move with the punches. Repeat ten (10) counts, work up to the point of fatigue. Inhale as you bring arms in, exhale as you bring arms out.

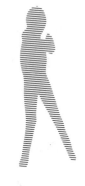

Deltoid, Trapezius, Triceps Muscles:

14.

Stand tall, knees relaxed, feet shoulder-width apart, pelvis in, abdomen tight, fists closed. Bring both arms out, shoulder level, now bend at the elbows and bring your fists in to touch under the armpits, then out again. Continue working arms in an in-out motion. Work movements slow and tight. Repeat ten (10) counts, work up to twenty (20) counts. Inhale as you bring arms in, exhale as you bring arms out.

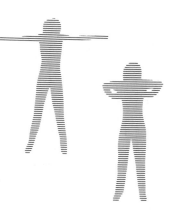

15.

Stand tall, knees relaxed, feet shoulder-width apart, abdomen tight, fists closed. Bring both arms out to your side, shoulder level. Now circle arms forward, using large circular motions. Relax body. Continue working arms in circular motion. Repeat ten (10) counts forward, then repeat in backward motion for ten (10) counts, breathing normally. (Do not use weights in this exercise.)

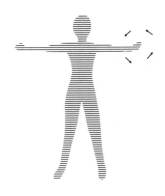

EXERCISES FOR THE ABDOMINAL MUSCLES AND LOWER BACK

The abdominal muscles are the hardest to work because we are working not just one, but many muscles. We work the entire length of the rectus abdominous and the muscles along the side of the abdomen (oblique muscles), as well as the muscles of the lower back.

Many people feel that they have a weak lower back, when in actuality they have weak abdominal muscles. When you strengthen the abdominals, the lower back is also strengthened.

It is important to keep a few rules in mind while you are working your abdominal muscles.

1. Keep the small of the lower back flat against the floor at all times.

2. Keep the knees bent at all times.

3. Always inhale as you come down, exhale as you bring your body up.

4. Hold the abdominals in tight at all times.

5. The movement is small, don't feel that you have to come up high, it is the tightness and the control that is important.

6. Never jerk your body upward, always use smooth flowing movements.

7. If at anytime you feel the muscles burning, relax for a moment then pick up the movement again.

   (This is with any exercise, not just the abdominals.)

8. Don't get discouraged, give your body time to adjust to these extra demands. Start slow and work up.

MORE EXERCISES FOR THE ABDOMINALS

(Rectus Abdominous):

1.
Lay on mat or blanket, lower back flat against mat, knees bent, abdomen tight, chin into chest, arms extended past knees, upper shoulders slightly off mat. With knees together, feet apart, reach past your knees with your hands. Continue pulling upper body upward in smooth flowing movement, keeping shoulders off mat. Repeat ten (10) counts, work up to twenty (20). Relax, inhale as you come down, exhale as you bring your body up.

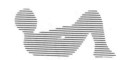

2.

In the same position, bring hands across chest. Continue pulling upper body upward in smooth flowing movement. Repeat ten (10) counts, work up to twenty (20). Inhale as you come down, exhale as you bring body up.

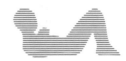

3a.

In same position as #1, bring hands behind head, elbows out, chin up. continue pulling upper body upward in smooth flowing movement, keeping shoulders off mat. Repeat ten (10) counts, work up to twenty (20). Inhale as you come down, exhale as you bring body up.

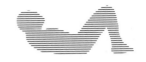

3b.

Bring knees into chest (one at a time), feet flexed. Place hands behind legs just below knees. Deeply inhale and then slowly exhale as you tighten hold around legs, till you feel buttocks slightly lifting off floor. Hold stretch for thirty (30) seconds. Relax.

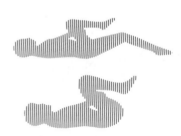

4.

Still lying on mat, bring knees into chest (one at a time), cross feet, lower back flat against mat, abdomen tight, chin into chest, arms extended past knees, upper shoulders slightly off mat. Reach past you knees with your hands. Continue pulling upper body upward in smooth flowing movement, keeping shoulders off mat. Repeat ten (10) counts, work up to twenty (20). Inhale as you come down, exhale as you bring your body up.

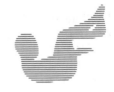

5.

In starting position, bring hands across chest. Continue pulling upper body upward in smooth flowing movement. Repeat ten (10) counts, work up to twenty (20). Relax, inhale as you come down, exhale as you bring your body up.

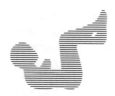

6.

In starting position, bring hands behind head, elbows out, chin up. Continue pulling upper body upward in smooth flowing movement. Repeat ten (10) counts, work up to twenty (20). Inhale as you come down, exhale as you bring your body up.

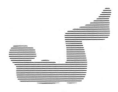

7.

Lying on mat, bring legs straight up, knees slightly relaxed, abdomen tight, chin into chest, arms extended past knees, upper shoulders slightly off mat. Reach past your knees with your hands. Continue pulling upper body upward in smooth flowing movement. Repeat ten (10) counts, work up to twenty (20). Inhale as you come down, exhale as you bring body up.

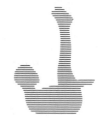

8.

In same position, bring hands across chest. Continue pulling upper body upward in smooth flowing movement. Repeat ten (10) counts, work up to twenty (20). Inhale as you come down, exhale as you bring body up.

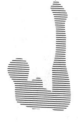

9a.

In same position, bring hands behind head, elbows out, chin up. Continue pulling upper body upward in smooth flowing movement. Repeat ten (10) counts, work up to twenty (20). Inhale as you come down, exhale as you bring body up.

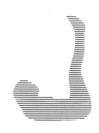

9b.

Bring knees into chest (one at a time), feet flexed. Place hands behind legs, just below knees. Inhale deeply, then slowly exhale as you tighten hold around back of legs, till you feel buttocks slightly lifting off floor. Hold stretch for thirty (30) seconds, relax.

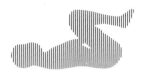

Side of Abdomen and Lower Back

(External Obliques):

10.

Lying on mat, bring knees into chest (one at a time). Lower back flat against mat, abdomen tight, chin slightly into chest, hands behind your head, upper shoulders slightly off mat. Keeping upper body in fixed position, bring left leg up, knee bent, left foot flat against floor. On right foot, point toe as you extend leg out. Now, as you bring right leg into body, knee bent, bring elbow of your left arm to touch right knee. Continue this half bicycle-type motion, in-out and elbow over to touch right knee. Repeat ten (10) counts with toe pointed, then ten (10) counts with foot flexed. Repeat for other leg. Inhale as you extend leg out, exhale as you bring knee in and elbow over.

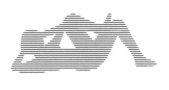

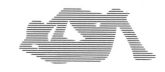

11a.

Lying on mat, bring knees into chest one at a time). Pull feet into right side of your body, letting your knees fall over to the left side of your body. Stretch you upper body toward right side. Hands behind your head, chin in. Concentrate on pulling upper body upward, using your left side abdominal muscles (obliques). Make each movement smooth. Repeat ten (10) counts, work up to twenty (20). Repeat for right side abdominal muscles. Relax, inhale as you come down, exhale as you bring body up.

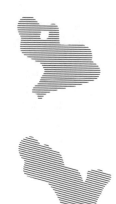

11b.

Bring knees into chest (one at a time), feet flexed. Place hands behind legs, just below knees. Inhale deeply and then slowly exhale as you tighten hold around back of legs, till you feel buttocks slightly lifting off floor. Hold stretch for thirty (30) seconds, relax.

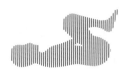

12.

Turn over onto stomach. Place hands even with chest, legs outstretched. Inhale deeply then slowly exhale. Lift upper body, keeping hips down, chin up. Hold stretch for fifteen (15) seconds, relax. Repeat one (1) time. Relax.

(This stretch helps to release the abdominal muscles you have worked so hard.)

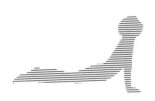

EXERCISES FOR THE HIPS, THIGHS AND BUTTOCKS

(Starting Position—Lay on left side and work right leg first.)

Outer Thigh:

1.

Lying on mat on your left side, rest your head in your left hand, bring left knee into body; resting on mat to support your lower back. Bring right knee into chest, foot flexed, right knee facing straight ahead, then extend leg out. Continue working right leg in an in-out motion, keeping foot flexed at all times. Repeat ten (10) counts. Inhale as you bring knee in, exhale as you extend leg out. Note: Body should be in a straight line with hips square.

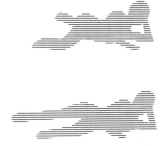

2.

In starting position, bring right knee into chest, foot flexed, this time with right knee facing straight upward, then extend leg out. Continue working right leg in an up-out motion, keeping foot flexed at all times. Repeat ten (10) counts. Inhale as you bring knee in, exhale as you extend leg out.

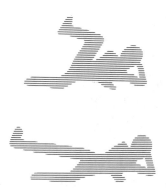

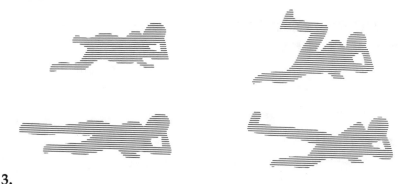

3.

In starting position; combine movements of exercises 1 and 2. Bring right knee to chest, foot flexed, with right knee facing straight ahead, then extend leg out, now work with right knee facing straight upward, then extend leg out. Continue working right leg in an in-out, up-out motion, keeping foot flexed at all times. Repeat ten (10) counts. Inhale as you bring knee in, exhale as you extend leg out.

4.

In starting position; extend right leg out, knee locked, foot flexed. Now lift right leg up about one foot off floor, do not allow top leg to touch bottom leg as you slowly squeeze buttocks back down, continue to lift leg in an up-down squeezing motion.
Repeat for twenty (20) counts.

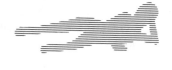

5.

In starting position; bring right leg all the way up, place right hand around calf to support leg as you flex and point foot, for one (1) count. Repeat ten (10) counts. Inhale as you point foot, exhale as you flex.

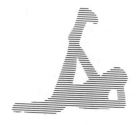

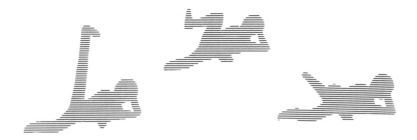

6.

In starting position; (a) bring right leg all the way up, foot flexed; (b) bend right leg at the knee into body; (c) with knee bent, bring bent leg all the way over, now bring leg back up to position (b) (bend right leg at the knee into body) with knee facing straight (d) then straighten leg all the way up to position (a) and bring back down to floor, do not allow top leg to touch bottom leg. This is one count. Repeat entire exercise for ten (10) counts. Inhale as you bring leg up, exhale as you bring leg over.

7.

In starting position, bend right leg at the knee into body. Bring bent leg all the way over as you squeeze buttocks tight, then up again. Keeping knee bent, continue lifting bent leg in an up-over squeezing motion. Repeat ten (10) counts. Inhale as you bring leg up, exhale as you squeeze bent leg over.

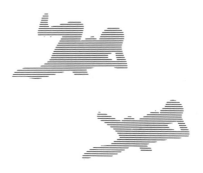

NOTE: Remember to keep foot in flexed position at all times. Do not let your hip rock over, use the muscles in the thigh and buttocks by pretending there is a wall against your back and you can't rock your hip.

Back of Thigh and Buttocks

(Hamstrings and Gluteus Maximus)

8.

Lying on mat, still on your left side,
with your left knee into body, resting
on mat to support your lower back.
Roll your body slightly over so that
your right hip and chest are facing
the floor. Rest your upper body on
your elbows, your chin in your
hand. Lift your right leg up and
back, toe pointed. Leg should be
lifted about two feet off floor, do
not allow top leg to touch floor as
you bring it back down. Continue
lifting leg in an up-down motion,
repeat twenty (20) counts. Then flex
foot and continue lifting leg up and down, repeat twenty (20)
counts. Inhale as you bring leg down, exhale as you lift leg.

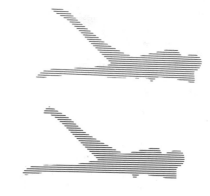

9.

Turn body over on to stomach, resting chin in your hands.
Lift right leg up about two feet, toes pointed,
continue slowly lifting leg in an
up-down motion, repeat twenty (20)
counts. Flex foot and
continue lifting leg in
up-down motion,
repeat twenty (20)
counts. Inhale as
you bring leg
down, exhale
as you
lift leg.

10.

Turn body on left side, head resting

10.

Turn body on left side, head resting in left hand, with left knee bent into body and resting on mat to support your lower back. Right leg lifted up, straight out, with foot flexed, now bend right knee back into body towards right buttocks, and extend leg out again. Continue working leg in an in-out kicking motion, repeat twenty (20) counts. Inhale as you bring leg in, exhale as you extend leg out.

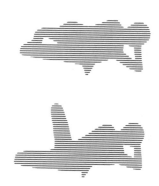

Inner Thigh

(Abductors):

(Starting position—Turn body on right side, right arm extended all the way out, head resting on arm. Body should be in straight line with hips square—bend left knee in and over right leg, resting on mat.)

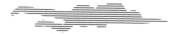

11.

Turn body on right side, right arm extended all the way out, head resting on arm. Body should be in straight line with hips square—bend left knee in and over right leg, resting on mat. Right foot pointed, right knee facing straight out to the side (or forward). Right leg should be lifted about one (1) inch off floor. Continue lifting right leg in an up-down motion, making sure knee is

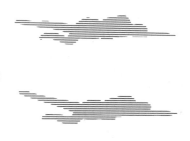

facing straight ahead, pressing leg down tightly (not upward). Repeat ten (10) counts. Inhale as you bring leg down, exhale as you lift.

continue to left right leg in up-press
down motion with knee pointed
straight out to the side (or forward).
Repeat ten (10) counts, inhale as you
bring leg down, exhale as you lift.

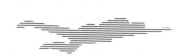

13.

In starting position, combine exercises 11 and 12. Point toes as you lift

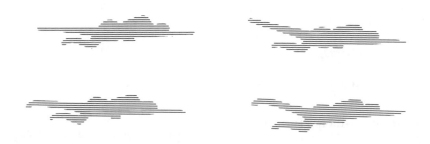

right leg, then flex foot as you lift (this is one count). Repeat for ten (10)
counts. Inhale as you press leg down, exhale as you lift.

14.

In starting position, toes pointed on
right leg, knee still facing straight out
to the side (or forward), hold right leg
up, holding tight, just above the floor,
hold up for ten (10) counts. Now with
toes still pointed lift leg from a raised
position in an up-down motion.
Repeat ten (10) counts.

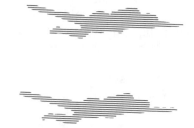

15.

In starting position, flex foot of right

leg, knee facing straight out to the
side (or forward). Hold right leg
up, holding tight, just above floor,
hold up for ten (10) counts. Now
with foot still flexed, lift leg from a
lifted position in an up-down motion.
Repeat ten (10) counts. Inhale as
you bring leg down, exhale as you lift.

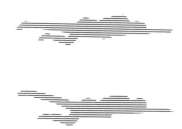

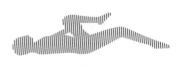

16.

Lay on your back with your head
resting straight. Extend your left
leg out, bend right knee into chest,
place right arm behind your knee
as you gently pull leg back as far
as you can. Hold stretch for
thirty (30) seconds, relax.
Breathe normally.

NOTE: This stretch helps to release the muscles you have worked so
hard.

*Shake both legs out and repeat the entire routine for the other side.
Lie on your right side and work your left leg.*

BUTTOCK TUCKS

(GLUTEOUS MAXIMUS)

(Starting Position—Lying on your back, feet parallel, shoulder-width
apart, abdomen tight, arms resting alongside your body.)

1.

Lying on your back, feet parallel,
shoulder-width apart, abdomen tight,

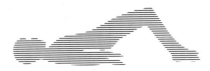

1.

Lying on your back, feet parallel, shoulder-width apart, abdomen tight, arms resting alongside your body. Lower back tight against mat, lift buttocks slightly off mat, now squeeze buttocks as tight as you can, then relax slightly, continue squeezing and relaxing motion, repeat ten (10) counts. Inhale as you relax; exhale as you squeeze.

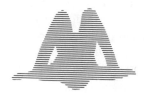

2.

In starting position, lower back tight against the mat. Abdomen tight, turn feet out to the side, let your legs drop open, with buttocks slightly lifted off mat, continue to squeeze and relax buttocks. Repeat ten (10) counts. Inhale as you relax, exhale as you squeeze.

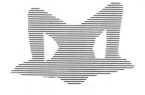

3.

In starting position, bring feet together, bring right foot over to rest against left leg, just below knee area. With lower back tight against mat, abdomen tight, buttocks slightly lifted off mat, continue to squeeze and relax buttocks. Repeat ten (10) counts, repeat for the other leg. Inhale as you relax, exhale as you squeeze.

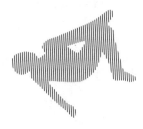

4.

In starting position, bring both legs
closer together, with lower back tight
against floor, abdomen tight, buttocks
slightly lifted off mat, feet on tiptoes,
continue to squeeze and relax buttocks.
Repeat ten (10) counts.

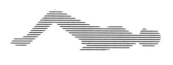

Now with feet resting on your heels, continue to squeeze and relax
buttocks, repeat ten (10) counts.
Relax.

Now with feet flat against floor, knees together, continue to squeeze and
relax buttocks. Repeat ten (10) counts. Relax.

Relaxing Lower Back:

5.

Lying on your back relax the body,
extend left leg out, bring right knee
into body, foot flexed. Place hands in
back of leg just below knee. Inhale
deeply then slowly exhale as you bring
leg tighter into body. Hold stretch for
thirty (30) seconds. Relax.

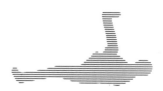

5a.

Bring right foot into body, with left
hand hold onto right ankle, place
right hand in back of right knee.
Inhale deeply then exhale slowly as
you bring leg tighter into body,
holding firmly to foot and back of
leg. Hold stretch for thirty (30)
seconds, relax.

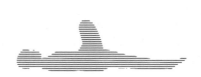

5b.

Extend leg all the way up,
place hands around calf to
support leg. Flex and point
foot for four (4)
counts, relax.

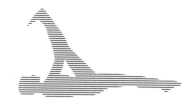

5c.

Bend right knee into chest, place right
arm behind your knee as you gently pull
leg back as far as you can. Hold stretch
for thirty (30) seconds, relax. Repeat
entire stretch for other leg, relax. Breathe
normally. Go into cool down.

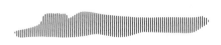

COOL DOWN

1.

Lying on mat, extend legs out
one at a time. Bring arms over
your head, resting on mat.
Inhale deeply as you stretch
body in opposite directions,
slowly exhale as you relax body.

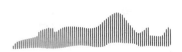

2.

Flex your feet, arms extended over
head, resting on mat. Move legs
as in walking motion, stretching
arms out in opposite directions.
Continue walking motion for
thirty (30) seconds. Deeply inhale
as you bring legs slightly into body,
slowly exhale as you extend legs.

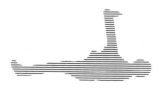

3.

Bring both knees into chest, (one leg at a time) with feet flexed. Place hands behind legs, just below the knees. Inhale deeply then slowly exhale, while tightening hold around legs till you feel buttocks slightly lifting off mat. Hold the stretch for thirty (30) seconds, relax.

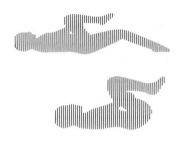

4.

Lying on mat with knees bent, lift upper body up to a sitting position with legs extended straight out from body. Inhale as you bring your hands over your head, slowly exhale as you bring your body forward, arms outstretched to grab your ankles. Hold head in a natural position (not held too high or low), and hold stretch for thirty (30) seconds. Relax.

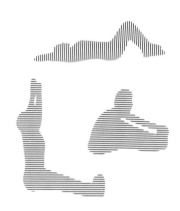

5.

Sitting, extend legs out to the side as far apart as you can comfortably. Inhale as you lean your body over to the right, exhale as you bring your left arm over your head stretching to the right, with you right arm extended out along your right leg, holding your right ankle to support lower back. Hold this position for thirty (30) seconds. (Do not bounce, just hold an easy stretch), then turn your body into leg and hold for three (3) seconds. Breathe normally. On lifting, push up using your right hand on your right ankle to support lower back. Slowly bring your body up in center position. Repeat for other side.

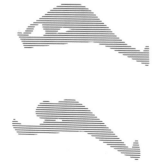

6.

Bring legs together, legs extended
straight out from body, inhale as
you lean your body forward. Slowly
exhale as your arms stretch out to
grab your ankles. Hold head in a
natural position (not too high or too
low). Hold the stretch for thirty (30)
seconds. Relax.

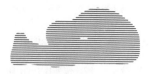

CHAPTER 10

Recipes for Health

The Main Course

BAKED HEN

1 Hen (6 to 8 lbs.)
1 Tsp. each black pepper, red pepper, sea salt, and garlic powder

Bird should be stuffed, if desired, just before baking. Either Cornbread or Brown Rice Dressing can be used. (If cornbread dressing is used it is not necessary to cook portion used before stuffing.

Season bird well, spoon in stuffing, filling cavity but do not pack. Place in deep pan, cover and bake at 325 degrees for 3½ to 4 hours. Adjust baking time if using a larger or smaller hen.

Serving Size ....   3.3 oz.
Calories 160
Protein 26
Carbs. 0
Fat 5

BAKED TURKEY

1 Turkey (12 to 16 lbs.)
1 tsp. each black pepper, red pepper, sea salt and garlic powder

Bird should be stuffed, if desired, just before baking. Either Cornbread or Brown Rice Dressing can be used. (If cornbread dressing is used it is not necessary to cook portion used before stuffing.

Season bird well, spoon in stuffing, filling cavity generously but do not pack. Place in deep pan, cover and bake at 325 degrees for 4½ to 5½ hours. Adjust baking time if using a larger or smaller turkey.

If smoked turkey is preferred, smoke according to instructions on smoker, or have bird smoked by a professional smokehouse.

Serving Size . . . .   3 oz.
Calories 375
Protein 26
Carbs. 0
Fat 5

CAJUN CHICKEN GUMBO

1 — 3 lb. fryer (cut up and skinned)
1 cup onions (chopped fine)
12 cups water
1 Tbsp. gumbo filé
1 cup green onions (chopped)
Salt, black pepper, and red pepper to taste
Roux (see following recipe)

In a large pot, bring water to a boil. Add roux (see recipe). Stir in all ingredients except filé and green onions. Simmer until chicken is tender. Add remaining ingredients and serve over brown rice.

Serving Size .... 1 cup
Calories ....186 (total calories with roux)
Protein 5
Carbs. 9
Fat 13

ROUX

1 cup unbleached flour
½ cup oil
1 cup cold water

In a heavy skillet, heat oil and add flour. Slowly cook mixture over low heat until dark, stirring continuously for about 45 minutes or until oil separates from flour. Be sure roux is dark enough. When roux is done, add water slowly, mixing well. Add to large pot of boiling water. Mix in well.

From this basic roux, chicken or seafood gumbo can be made by following the previous recipe.

Serving Size .... Makes approximately 2 cups
Calories 1356
Fat 110

CHICKEN QUICHE

1 Whole Wheat Pie Shell (see recipe)
1 cup cooked chicken or turkey (cut up into bite-size pieces)
1 cup shredded Swiss and Cheddar cheese
⅓ cup chopped onion
4 eggs
2 cups Lowfat milk
1 tsp. sea salt
½ tsp. thyme
½ tsp. each black pepper and red pepper

Prepare pastry. Sprinkle chicken, cheese, and onion into pie shell. Beat eggs slightly, beat in remaining ingredients. Pour into pie shell.

Bake uncovered in 425 degree oven for 15 minutes. Reduce oven temperature to 300 degrees. Bake uncovered until knife inserted halfway between center and edge comes out clean, or about 30 minutes. Let stand for 10 minutes before cutting.

Serving Size . . . . 6 servings
Calories 232
Protein 20
Carbs. 6
Fat 14

ALMOND CHICKEN

½ cup slivered almonds
2½ cups cooked chicken
4 Tbsp. olive oil
¼ cup flour
¼ cup white raisins
½ cup sliced mushrooms
1 cup chicken stock
Dash each salt and pepper

Melt half the olive oil in a large skillet. Sauté mushrooms about 2 minutes. Add rest of olive oil, flour, salt, and pepper to taste. Add raisins and chicken. Cook about 10 minutes, then add stock and simmer 10 minutes.

Serve topped with almonds over rice or toast.

Serving Size 4
Calories 358
Protein 12
Carbs. 14
Fat 13

CHICKEN SOUP

1 — 3 lb. whole chicken
8 cups cold water
2 medium onions
2 stalks celery
3 carrots chopped
5 sprigs fresh parsley
1 bay leaf
¼ tsp. thyme
6 whole peppercorns
2 tsp. salt

Place chicken in pot with water, breast side down. Add one onion cut into quarters, one stalk celery cut into 2" lengths, parsley, bay leaf, thyme, peppercorns and salt. Bring slowly to a boil, lower heat and simmer for 1 hour. Remove chicken from pot and set aside to cool. Strain broth and return to pot.

Chop remaining onion and celery. Add to broth along with carrots and additional seasonings. Bring to a boil, then simmer 15 minutes. Add meat and simmer 5 minutes more. Serve hot. Garnish with parsley. For a heartier soup, add rice or cubed potatoes along with other chopped vegetables.

Serving Size   4
Calories 774
Protein 70
Carbs. 12
Fat 53

CHICKEN ROSEMARY

2½ lbs. chicken
½ cup whole wheat flour
1 tsp. sea salt
2 tsp. crushed rosemary
⅛ tsp. pepper

Chicken breasts, drumsticks, or wings are fine to use. Mix flour, rosemary, salt and pepper in a shallow bowl. Wash chicken and coat with flour mixture. Let coated parts dry for about ½ hour. Bake chicken in a 350 degree oven for 1 hour.

Serving Size 4
Calories 622
Protein 55
Carbs. 11
Fat 38

CHICKEN AND MUSHROOMS

3 lb. chicken
1 lb. sliced mushroom
2 cloves chopped garlic
1 sliced onion
6 Tbsp. olive oil
1 Tbsp. butter
2 Tbsp. water
¼ tsp. crushed basil
½ tsp. crushed tarragon
Dash each salt and pepper

Cut chicken into serving pieces. Wash and pat dry. Season with salt and pepper. In a skillet heat butter, garlic, and ⅔ of oil. Brown chicken on both sides (about 10 minutes). Lower heat and continue cooking for 25 minutes.

In separate skillet, heat 2 Tbsp. oil. Sauté onions until clear, about 5 minutes. Add mushrooms and 2 Tbsp. water, simmer 10 minutes; add to chicken.

Cover and simmer chicken 15 minutes. Heat to boiling for 1 minute. Serve hot.

Serving Size 4
Calories 976
Protein 70
Carbs. 18
Fat 77

CHICKEN AND RICE SOUP

1 cup brown rice
¾ cup wild rice
1 cup diced chicken
2 cups chopped celery leaves and stalks
1½ cup sliced mushrooms
1 medium cubed potato
1 large sliced pepper
1 pinch crushed red pepper
2 large bay leaves
1 tsp. celery seed
¼ tsp. oregano
1 tsp. fresh parsley
1 tsp. dried spinach
3 cloves crushed garlic

Place all ingredients in a large soup pot and cook over low heat for about 1½hours.

Serving Size 4
Calories 325
Protein 12
Carbs. 64
Fat 3

PARMESAN BUTTERED FISH

1 lb. trout (filet and cut into small pieces)
½ cup butter
2 Tbsp. lemon juice
½ cup parmesan cheese
paprika and pepper to taste

Lay fish in deep baking dish, set aside. Melt butter in pan until slightly brown. Add lemon juice and mix well. Pour ¼ cup butter mixture over fish. Bake at 375 degrees until fish turns slightly white, about 15 minutes. Do not overcook.

Remove from oven, add parmesan cheese and remaining butter to fish. Sprinkle with paprika and pepper. Return to oven, bake about 5 minutes or until cheese is melted. Garnish with parsley and lemon slices.

Bass, perch, bream or other small fish fillet can be substituted with excellent results.

```
Serving Size  . . . . . . . .   3 oz.
Calories  . . . . . . . . .135
Protein  . . . . . . . . . .22
Carbs.  . . . . . . . . . . .0
Fat  . . . . . . . . . . . . . .4
```

FISH WITH TAHINI SAUCE

1 Tbsp. olive oil
1 large minced onion
1 lb. fresh catfish filets
Sea salt (optional)
1 clove minced garlic
2 Tbsp. tahini sauce
¼ cup fresh lemon juice

Heat the olive oil in a large skillet. Sauté the onion over moderate heat until soft but not brown. Set aside.

Heat oven to 350 degrees. Spread the onions in a baking dish large enough to hold the filets in one layer. Add the filets. Sprinkle with a little salt if desired. Bake the fish and onions for 10 minutes.

While the fish is baking, crush the garlic, stir in the tahini and lemon juice and mix well. Spread the fish with the tahini mixture and bake 10 to 20 minutes more or until fish flakes easily with a fork.

Serving Size 4
Calories 162
Protein 21
Carbs. 4
Fat 7

OKRA GUMBO

2 lbs. fresh okra — sliced thin
¼ cup oil
2 cups onions, chopped
2 large bell peppers, chopped
3 cloves garlic, minced
2 fresh tomatoes, skinned and chopped
½ cup tomato puree
2½ cups water
Salt, black pepper, and red pepper to taste

In a deep, heavy pot heat oil and add okra, onions, bell peppers, and garlic. Cook slowly over medium heat, stirring frequently, making sure that okra does not stick and burn. Cook until okra has completely lost its gummy texture (about 1 hour).

Add water, tomatoes, and tomato puree. Cook over medium to low heat 1½ hours. Serve over brown rice.

Serving Size .... 1 cup
Calories 110
Protein 1
Carbs. 4
Fat 7

PIZZA CRUST

1 cup warm water
2 pkg. dry yeast
½ tsp. salt
2½ cups whole wheat flour

Mix water with yeast and salt. Add flour, mixing well with an electric mixer. Knead a few times. Place in oiled pan, turning mixture once to oil both sides. Set in a warm place to rise until doubled in size (about 1 hour). Punch down dough, knead a few times. Separate into two balls. Pat out onto a 12 inch pizza pan, making sure that the crust is thin. For a crispy crust, bake in a 350 degree oven for 5 minutes. Use following recipe for sauce.

PIZZA SAUCE

½ cup water
2 fresh turkey breast tenderloins — chopped up in food processor
1 tsp. fennel seed
1 tsp. rosemary leaves
1 tsp. bay leaves powder
1 tsp. Italian seasoning
1 tsp. oregano
1 tsp. parsley flakes
½ tsp. basil leaves
½ tsp. garlic powder
1 — 12 oz. can Contadina Tomato Paste
1 — 16 oz. can stewed tomatoes (from health food store)
1 cup water
½ cup chopped onion
½ cup chopped bell pepper
1 small onion (sliced thin)
1 small bell pepper (sliced thin)
1 cup sliced mushrooms
8 oz. shredded Mozzarella cheese
8 oz. shredded Cheddar cheese

In large skillet brown turkey with chopped onion, bell pepper, and seasonings. Add tomato paste, stewed tomatoes, and water. Cook over medium fire, stirring occasionally until bubbling. Pour ½ mixture into each pizza crust. Top with sliced onion, bell pepper, and mushrooms.

Cover with shredded cheeses. Bake at 350 degrees for 20 minutes.

```
Yield  . . . . . . . . . . . . .   2 — 12 inch pizzas — 16 slices
Serving Size  . . . . . . . .   1 slice
Calories  . . . . . . . . .155
Protein  . . . . . . . . . .8.4
Carbs.  . . . . . . . . . . .15
Fat  . . . . . . . . . . . . . .5.3
```

LASAGNA

1 box 10 oz. DeBoles Substitute Curly Lasagna
1 — 20 oz. can Spicy chili (No meat — Natural Touch brand from health food store)
1 Tbsp. olive oil
1 cup chopped onions
1 medium bell pepper — chopped
¼ tsp. garlic powder
1 cup Dannon Non-Fat Yogurt
1 cup (1 oz.) shredded natural cheddar cheese

Boil lasagna in about four quarts of water. Drop lasagna strips one at a time into boiling water. Cook 7 to 10 minutes, drain and set aside.

Saute onions, bell pepper, and garlic powder in olive oil until clear. Add spicy chili and yogurt. Simmer over low heat, stirring occasionally for 15 minutes.

In a 13" X 9" pan, arrange one layer of lasagna, overlapping the edges. Spoon ½ of mixture over noodles, sprinkle with ½ cup of cheddar cheese, Repeat for next layer, top with remaining cheese. Bake at 350 degrees for 20 minutes.

Serving Size .... 9 (3"x 4")
Calories 295
Protein 11
Carbs. 32
Fat 16

VEGETABLE SOUP

6 cups water
3 stalks celery
2 medium onions (approx. 2 cups)
1 tsp. salt
pepper (to taste)
2 Tbsp. instant chicken soup mix (no sugar from health food store)
2 Tbsp. instant onion soup mix (no sugar from health food store)
2 medium carrots
1 can tomato sauce (15 oz. no sugar)
2 fresh tomatoes (skinned and sliced)
1 small zucchini (sliced thin)
1 cup frozen English peas (no sugar)

Mix all ingredients into a large pot and cook over low heat for about 1½ hours.

Serving Size . . . .   12 — 1 cup servings
Calories 36
Protein 2
Carbs. 7
Fat 1

CORN & POTATO SOUP

8 cups water
3 red potatoes (approx. 1 lb.)
3 ears fresh corn (cut off cob)
1 cup chopped onions
1 Tbsp. Vegetarian Style Chicken Cream Soup Mix (Mayacamas brand)
½ tsp. garlic powder
Salt and pepper to taste

Place all ingredients in deep heavy pot. Bring to boil over medium heat. Lower heat, cover, and simmer for approximately 1 hour.

Serving Size .... approx. 4 — 1 cup servings
Calories 140
Protein 6
Carbs. 33
Fat ....trace

SPAGHETTI ALTONNO

½ cup chopped bell pepper
½ cup chopped onion
2 — 7 oz. cans tuna
2 — 8 oz. cans tomato sauce
½ cup water
2 tsp. sea salt
1 tsp. oregano
½ tsp. garlic powder
⅓ cup olive oil
⅛tsp. pepper
1 pkg. thin whole wheat spaghetti

Boil whole grain spaghetti. Heat oil in a large skillet. Add chopped bell pepper and onion and sauté until tender.

Stir in tuna fish, tomato sauce, water salt, oregano, garlic powder, and pepper. Cook until thoroughly heated about 5 to 10 minutes. Pour sauce over cooked spaghetti. If desired, sprinkle with grated cheese.

Serves 4
Calories 594
Protein 31
Carbs. 88
Fat 18

Vegetable and Side Dishes

STEAMED CABBAGE

1 small cabbage (diced)
¼ tsp. garlic powder
½ cup onions (chopped)
Salt (to taste)
1 cup water

In an Hitachi rice cooker, add water, put in steamer plate. Add cabbage, onions, garlic powder and salt. Set cooker.

Instead of an Hitachi rice cooker, a regular steamer can be used. Cook for 30 minutes.

Serving Size .... ½ cup
Calories 24
Protein 1
Carbs. 4
Fat .... trace

NAVY BEANS

1 cup dried navy beans (soak in water overnight, refrigerate.)
1 cup onions (chopped)
½ cup celery (chopped)
3 cloves garlic (minced)
4 cups water
Salt (to taste)

Combine ingredients in large covered saucepan. Cook over medium heat until beans are tender, about 2 hours. More water may be added if needed. Serve over brown rice.

Yield .... Approx. 8 cups
Serving Size .... 1 cup
Calories 39
Protein 2
Carbs. 7
Fats 0

STRING BEANS AND POTATOES

3 cups fresh snapped string beans
1 Tbsp. olive oil
1 cup onion (chopped)
3 cloves garlic (minced)
1 cup potatoes (diced)
½ cup water
Salt and pepper (to taste)

In heavy pot add onions, garlic, and potatoes with oil. Sauté about 5 minutes. Add beans and water. Cover and cook over medium heat for about ½ hour or until beans are tender.

```
Yield  ............  6 cups
Serving Size  ........  ½ cup
Calories  .........47
Protein  ...........1
Carbs.  ...........4
Fat  ..............1
```

CORN MAQUECHOI (MOCKSHOO)

4 ears tender corn
1 cup onions (chopped)
1 bell pepper (chopped)
3 cloves garlic (minced)
¼ cup oil
½ cup water

Shave off kernels from ears. Heat oil in heavy pot. Add all ingredients except water. Cook over low heat, stirring frequently for about 15 minutes. Add water, cover, and cook over low heat for 45 minutes.

Yield .... 8 cups
Serving Size .... ½ cup
Calories 52
Protein 1
Carbs. 1
Fat 1

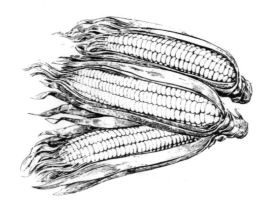

GREEN BEAN CASSEROLE

2 cups fresh green beans (snapped)
1 cup onions (chopped)
2 cloves garlic (minced)
½ cup water
2 Tbsp. Barths Instant Onion Soup Mix (from the health food store)
2 Tbsp. Mayacamas Chicken Style Soup Mix (from the health food store)
½ cup homemade bread crumbs (see recipe)
Salt, black pepper and red pepper (to taste)

Wash beans and place in deep baking dish; add onion, garlic, water and soup mixes. Mix well. top with bread crumbs, cover and bake at 350 degrees for 1 hour or until beans are tender.

```
Yield  . . . . . . . . . . . . .   Approx. 3 cups
Serving Size  . . . . . . . .   ½ cup
Calories  . . . . . . . . . .41
Protein . . . . . . . . . . . .1
Carbs.  . . . . . . . . . . . .8
Fat  . . . . . . . . . . . . . .1
```

CANDIED YAMS

3 medium-sized sweet potatoes
1 cup water
½ cup Sweet Cloud Rice Syrup (from the health food store)
½ tsp. cinnamon
½ tsp. ginger
¼ tsp. nutmeg
1 tsp. vanilla (no sugar kind)

Bake sweet potatoes at 350 degrees until tender, about 1½ hours. Peel and dice, place in deep baking dish, sprinkle with spices, set aside.

In heavy pot bring water and rice syrup to boil; lower heat and cook until mixture forms a hard ball (when dropped into a cup of cold water, mixture forms a ball). Remove from fire, add vanilla, pour over yams.

Bake at 350 degrees uncovered for 30 minutes. May be topped with whipped cream if desired.

Yield	Approx 3 cups
Serving Size	½ cup
Calories 183	
Protein 1	
Carbs. 41	
Fat 0	

ORIENTAL VEGETABLES

½ cup sliced onions
1 cup sliced carrots
1 cup sliced cauliflower
1 cup sliced green beans
2 Tbsp. peanut oil
1 cup water
2 tsp. chicken broth
2 tsp. whole wheat flour
Pinch garlic

In skillet, heat oil and cook sliced green beans, cauliflower, carrots, and onions. Combine sauce ingredients: water, chicken broth, flour, and garlic powder. Add to cooked vegetables. Heat through until thickened. You can vary recipe by increasing onion or using ½ the amount needed for onions and replace it with celery.

Yield . . . . serves 4
Calories 105
Protein 2
Carbs. 9
Fat 6.5

ZUCCHINI SOUP

2 medium zucchini
¼ cup chopped onions
¾ cup cooked brown rice
1 quart homemade chicken broth
1 tsp. curry powder
½ tsp. dijon mustard
¼ cup nonfat yogurt

Simmer zucchini, onion, and strained chicken broth in soup pot for 15 minutes. Add cooked rice. Puree in blender, adding curry powder, mustard, and yogurt to taste. Eat either warm or cold.

```
Yield  . . . . . . . . . . . . .   serves 4
Calories  . . . . . . . . .320
Protein  . . . . . . . . . .7.5
Carbs.  . . . . . . . . . . .46
Fat  . . . . . . . . . . . . .2.75
```

WATERCRESS SOUP

2 bunches chopped watercress
12 ozs. chopped potatoes
1 medium chopped onion
5 cups vegetable stock
bouquet garni
1 pinch sea salt
1 pinch cayenne pepper

Combine all ingredient. Bring to boil, simmer until vegetables are cooked but still slightly crisp.

Allow to cool. Remove bouquet garni. Chill before serving.

```
Yield  . . . . . . . . . . . . . .   Serves 4
Calories  . . . . . . . . .213
Protein . . . . . . . . . . . .6
Carbs.   . . . . . . . . . . .45
Fat   . . . . . . . . . . . . . . .0
```

SQUASH SOUP WITH TOFU

1 lb. squash/pumpkin, cut into 1" pieces
2 medium sliced onions
¼ tsp. cinnamon
¼ tsp. nutmeg
2 cloves minced garlic
4 Tbsp. miso (soybean soup from Health Food Store)
12 oz. tofu
3 Tbsp. chopped parsley
3 Tbsp. ground sesame seeds

Set aside tofu. In large sauce pan add all the other ingredients and bring to boil. Lower heat and simmer for about 5 to 8 minutes.

Cut tofu into bite size pieces. Add to soup and simmer for 5 more minutes. May be served over brown rice.

Yield . . . . Serves 4
Calories 194.5
Protein 10
Carbs. 24
Fat 1

AVOCADO STUFFED TOMATOES

4 large tomatoes
1 peeled avocado
½ cup chopped oat bran
½ cup chopped celery
2 Tbsp. parsley
2 Tbsp. lemon juice
1 pinch red pepper

Slice ½ inch off the top of each tomato, remove and finely chop pulp and tops. Drain the shells.

Combine tomato, other vegetables, and remaining ingredients. Mix well. Spoon into tomatoes and chill.

Yield . . . .   Serves 4
Calories 137
Protein 3.5
Carbs. 13.5
Fat 5

TOMATO PROVENCALE

2 whole tomatoes
1 Tbsp. chopped parsley
2 Tbsp. bread crumbs
1 Tbsp. olive oil
¼ tsp. salt
1 clove crushed garlic
pepper to taste

Cut tomatoes in half crosswise and remove seeds. Heat oil in skillet and sauté the tomatoes (cut side down) about 3 minutes. Turn and sprinkle with salt and pepper, sauté for 3 more minutes. Add garlic and bread crumbs; simmer until tomatoes are tender.

Place tomatoes on a heated serving dish and sprinkle with parsley.

Yield .... Serves 4
Calories 42
Protein 85
Carbs. 8
Fat 4

SAUTEED BROCCOLI

2 lbs. fresh broccoli
½ cup water
¼ cup peanut oil
2 cloves minced garlic
1 tsp. salt
⅛ tsp. pepper

Wash broccoli. Split ends of large stalks lengthwise or quarter, depending on the size. Place in a large skillet. Sprinkle with water, peanut oil, garlic, salt, and pepper. Cover tightly; cook over very low heat for 20 to 30 minutes, or until stalks are tender. Turn broccoli several times during cooking.

Yield .... Serves 4
Calories 168
Protein 4.5
Carbs. 8
Fat 14

ONION SOUP

6 large sliced onions
6 Tbsp. butter
6 cups fresh beef stock
1 Tbsp. ground whole wheat flour
4 slices french bread cut ¾" thick (no sugar added, homemade)
1 cup grated swiss cheese

Spread french bread with ⅓ of the butter; toast until brown and set aside.

In soup pot melt remaining butter. Add onions and sauté until tender. Add stock. Add salt and pepper to taste. Add flour and mix until smooth. Simmer for about 15 minutes. Pour in separate serving bowls and place toasted bread on top. Sprinkle with swiss cheese and broil until light brown.

```
Yield  . . . . . . . . . . . . . .   Serves 4
Calories  . . . . . . . . .470
Protein . . . . . . . . . .14
Carbs.  . . . . . . . . . .35
Fat  . . . . . . . . . . . . .21
```

NOODLES ROMANOFF

6 oz. whole grain noodles
1 cup sour cream
½ cup parmesan cheese
1 clove crushed garlic
1 Tbsp. butter
½ tsp. snipped chives
½ tsp. salt
dash pepper

Start by cooking noodles as package directs. Stir together sour cream, half the cheese, chives, salt, pepper, and garlic in a bowl. Set aside.

Drain noodles and return to pan. Stir in butter. Fold in sour cream mixture. Place on a serving platter and sprinkle with the remaining cheese.

Yield . . . . Serves 4
Calories 361
Protein 14
Carbs. 32
Fat 4

LEEK SOUP

2 stalks sliced leek
1 Tbsp. butter
1 Tbsp. olive oil
½ tsp. salt
2 cups vegetable stock

Melt butter until foamy. Add olive oil and sliced leek. Lower heat and simmer for about 1½ minutes. Add homemade vegetable stock and salt to leeks. Bring to a boil. Remove from heat. Garnish with finely chopped parsley and serve.

Yield .... Serves 4
Calories 67.5
Protein 0
Carbs. 4.5
Fat 9

LENTIL SOUP

2 cups dried lentils
2 chopped carrots
1 chopped onion
1 stalk chopped celery
2 cloves crushed garlic
1 bay leaf
8 cups cold water
1 Tbsp. salt
1 tsp. pepper

Wash and sort lentils. Place in pot with water and bring to a boil. Cook uncovered, over medium heat about 20 minutes. Skim frequently. Add vegetables, garlic, and bay leaf. Bring to a boil, reduce heat and simmer about 45 minutes or until lentils are tender. Season with salt and pepper. Garnish with chopped parsley. Serve hot.

```
Yield  .............   Serves 4
Calories  .........380
Protein . . . . . . . . . . . .
Carbs.   ..........69
Fat   ..............0
```

ALMOND GARLIC SOUP

½ loaf homemade French bread
½ cup water
½ cup blanched almonds
3 cloves garlic
3 Tbsp. olive oil
2 tsp. vinegar
2 cups chilled chicken stock
dash sea salt
dash pepper
10 green grapes

Remove crust from bread and soak it in water. Place moist bread in food processor or blender along with almonds, garlic, oil, and vinegar; puree until smooth.

Add stock, season to taste and then chill. Serve in individual bowls over an ice cube. Garnish with green grapes.

```
Yield  . . . . . . . . . . . . .   Serves 4
Calories  . . . . . . . . .248
Protein  . . . . . . . . . .1.5
Carbs.  . . . . . . . . . . .4
Fat  . . . . . . . . . . . . .40
```

LEMON BROCCOLI

1 bundle broccoli
1 tsp. salt
¼ cup salad oil
½ clove minced garlic
2 tsp. lemon juice
6 cups boiling water

Prepare broccoli, wash and drain. Split stalks. Place in large saucepan with boiling water and salt. Cover and cook until tender, about 10 minutes. Drain. Heat garlic and oil in a small pan. Add broccoli; sprinkle with lemon juice and salt. Cook until broccoli is heated through.

Yield .... Serves 4
Calories 144
Protein 3
Carbs. 5
Fat 14

GAZPACHO

1 clove mashed garlic
1 peeled chopped onion
5 ripe peeled tomatoes
1 cup beef bouillon
3 Tbsp. olive oil
2 Tbsp. vinegar
2 Tbsp. chopped parsley
dash paprika
1 med. chopped green pepper
2 cuccumbers blended
1 cuccumber finely chopped

Combine garlic and onion in blender and blend until smooth. Add the remaining ingredients; cover the container and blend the mixture until it is smooth.

Chill soup thoroughly. Serve the following items in separate bowls with the soup: Cucumbers, green peppers, tomatoes, onions (all finely chopped), and croutons.

```
Yield  . . . . . . . . . . . . . .   Serves 4
Calories  . . . . . . . . .157
Protein . . . . . . . . . . . .8
Carbs.  . . . . . . . . . . .11
Fat  . . . . . . . . . . . . . .10
```

GARLIC SOUP

6 cloves garlic
4 cups chicken stock
2 Tbsp. olive oil
15 blanched almonds
2 slices cubed bread
1 tsp. salt
½ tsp. pepper
½ cup balled honeydew melon balls

Quickly fry almonds and blend or pound with garlic to make a paste.
Heat oil in sauce pan; add bread cubes and garlic paste. Stir and cook until cubes are light brown. Remove from pan and blend well. Add chicken stock, stirring thoroughly. Add salt and pepper. Puree in blender, then chill. Garnish with honeydew melon balls and an ice cube in each bowl.

Yield .... Serves 4
Calories 137
Protein 7
Carbs. 8
Fat 10.9

GINGER CARROT SOUP

½ tsp. minced ginger root
1 cloves minced garlic
½ tsp. olive oil
2½ cups sliced carrots
2 cups homemade chicken broth
¼ cup fresh lime juice
nonfat yogurt garnish

In a soup pot or large casserole, sauté ginger, garlic, and onion in olive oil until tender. Add strained chicken broth and simmer until carrots are tender, about 20 minutes. Add lime juice and puree soup in blender until smooth.

Serve warm or chilled with a large dollop of yogurt.

Yield .... Serves 4
Calories 54
Protein 4
Carbs. 7
Fat 2

GARDEN PEA SOUP

2 lbs. fresh peas
1 quart vegetable stock
1 tsp. light cream
1 tsp. chopped chives
1 chopped onion
1 pinch sea salt
1 pinch cayenne pepper

Shell peas, chop onions and add to boiling stock. Simmer 20 minutes or until peas are cooked. Remove from heat. Cool. Puree in blender. Add cream, chives, seasoning to taste.

```
Yield  .............  Serves 4
Calories .........120
Protein ............8
Carbs.  ...........21
Fat  ..............1
```

CUCUMBER SOUP

1 large peeled cucumber
2 cups chicken broth
1½ cup buttermilk
1 tsp. curry powder
1 tsp. fresh lemon juice
1 pinch salt
1 pinch pepper
½ tsp. chopped chives

Dice cucumber. Put all ingredients in blender. Blend until smooth. Store in refrigerator several hours or overnight.

Garnish each serving with cucumber slices and chopped chives. Serve with croutons and carrot sticks. Makes an excellent cold soup.

**NOTE: Make your own chicken stock.

Yield .... Serves 4
Calories 63
Protein 6
Carbs. 6
Fat 1

VEGETABLE CASSEROLE

1 cup chopped broccoli
1 cup chopped cauliflower
1 cup chopped summer squash
½ cup slivered almonds
1 cup shredded cheddar cheese
¼ tsp. garlic powder
salt & pepper to taste

Lightly steam vegetables in steamer until slightly tender. Place in oblong baking dish, season with garlic, salt, and pepper. Sprinkle almonds over vegetables, top with cheese. Bake 30 minutes at 350 degrees.

Yield . . . . Serves 6
Calories 150
Protein 8
Carbs. 4
Fat 11

CHILLED WATERCRESS SOUP

3 cups fresh beef stock
4 peeled sliced potatoes
1 cup diced onion
2 Tbsp. butter
2 bunches watercress
1 egg yolk
1 cup heavy cream
1 tsp. salt

Cook potatoes and onion in beef stock until potatoes are soft. Take leaves off watercress, wash and chop; sauté lightly in butter. Add to beef stock and gently simmer for 10 minutes.

Puree in blender or food processor, season to taste with salt and pepper. Beat egg yolk in bowl and add cream slowly while beating. Add to beef stock gently. Chill and serve very cold. Garnish with thin slices of apple.

Yield .... Serves 4
Calories 400
Protein 10
Carbs. 48
Fat 8

ASPARAGUS SOUP

1½ lbs. fresh asparagus
1 Tbsp. minced onion
1 tsp. sea salt
2 cups fresh chicken stock
1½ light cream
1 Tbsp. chopped parsley
dash salt
dash pepper
4 tsp. butter

Break off asparagus stalks where they snap easily.

Discard ends and wash tips thoroughly; cut into pieces and place in sauce pan with onion, salt, parsley, and 1 cup of chicken stock. Cover and boil gently until tender.

Reserve a few tips for a garnish. Put the rest in a food processor and puree until smooth. Place puree in a sauce pan, add remaining stock, cream and season to taste. Heat but do not boil.

Serve hot and garnish with tips and a dab of butter on top.

```
Yield  . . . . . . . . . . . . . .   Serves 4
Calories  . . . . . . . . .101
Protein . . . . . . . . . . .24
Carbs.  . . . . . . . . . . .20
Fat  . . . . . . . . . . . . . .5.5
```

BASIL TOMATOES

3 medium sliced tomatoes
2 Tbsp. olive oil
1 tsp. basil
1 tsp. vinegar
pinch salt
pinch pepper
pinch garlic powder

Combine oil, vinegar, basil, salt, and pepper. Add tomatoes and evenly coat. Add pinch garlic powder. Chill at least 2 hours.

Yield .... Serves 4
Calories 49
Protein 80
Carbs 4
Fat 3

RICE AND PEAS

1 cup rice
1 pkg. frozen peas
6 Tbsp. olive oil
⅓ cup minced onion
2 Tbsp. minced parsley
1 tsp. salt
2 Tbsp. parmesan cheese
2 cups water

Cook peas according to directions, drain well and set aside. In heavy sauce pan, sauté onions and parsley with ⅔ of the oil for about 5 minutes. Add rice and continue to sauté for 5 minutes.

Add water and bring to boil, reduce heat, cover and simmer for 15 minutes.

```
Yield  . . . . . . . . . . . . . .   Serves 4
Calories  . . . . . . . . .436
Protein . . . . . . . . . . .8
Carbs.  . . . . . . . . . .48
Fat  . . . . . . . . . . . . .21
```

CURRIED RICE

3 cups cooked brown rice
1 egg yolk
1 tsp. curry powder
1 chopped green pepper
¼ tsp. salt
¼ tsp. pepper
2 Tbsp. butter
¼ tsp. cayenne
1 chopped onion

Sauté onion and green pepper in butter until onion is tender. Stir in curry powder, slightly beaten egg, salt, pepper, and cayenne pepper. Mix into hot rice. Sprinkle with chopped olive if available.

```
Yield  . . . . . . . . . . . . . .   Serves 4
Calories  . . . . . . . . .612
Protein  . . . . . . . . . . .13
Carbs.  . . . . . . . . . . .23
Fat  . . . . . . . . . . . . . . .3
```

RISOTTO

1 cup uncooked brown rice
½ cup chopped onion
2 cubes chicken bouillon
¼ cup parmesan cheese
2 cups boiling water
¼ tsp. saffron
2 Tbsp. olive oil

Heat oil and sauté onion in a deep skillet. Add rice and sauté, stirring frequently until light brown. Add saffron. Dissolve bouillon in boiling water and pour over rice. Cover tightly and simmer until rice is tender, about 20 minutes. Stir in parmesan cheese when serving.

```
Yield  . . . . . . . . . . . . . .   Serves 4
Calories  . . . . . . .246.5
Protein . . . . . . . . . . . .9
Carbs.  . . . . . . . . . . .40
Fat  . . . . . . . . . . . . . .12
```

MEXICAN RICE

1 cup uncooked brown rice
1 Tbsp. olive oil
1 Tbsp. butter
1 clove garlic
¼ cup minced onion
1 tsp. salt
½ tsp. pepper
⅓ cup tomato sauce
2 cups water

In skillet heat oil and butter. Add rice and cook until light brown. Add onions and garlic and sauté until onion is tender. Add salt, pepper, tomato sauce, and water. Stir once or twice, cover and simmer 60 minutes. Do not stir or uncover. Fluff with fork when ready to serve.

```
Yield  . . . . . . . . . . . . . .   Serves 4
Calories  . . . . . . . . .246
Protein . . . . . . . . . . .4
Carbs.  . . . . . . . . . .40
Fat  . . . . . . . . . . . . . .7
```

PERFECT BROWN RICE

2 cups brown rice
3 cups water
1 tsp. olive oil
salt (to taste)

Place all ingredients in a heavy four quart pot, bring to a boil over medium heat. Lower heat to very low, cover and simmer until rice is tender, about 1 hour. Remove from heat, stir with a fork. Serve topped with butter or gravy.

Yield	Approx. 6 cups
Serving Size	½ cup
Calories 29	
Protein 42	
Carbs. 5	
Fat 2	

CORNBREAD DRESSING

2 chicken breasts, skinned
8 cups water
6 boiled eggs
2 Tbsp. Mayacamas Chicken Style Soup Mix
¼ cup olive oil
1 cup chopped onions
1 cup chopped bell pepper
1 cup chopped celery
4 cloves minced garlic
1 ½ tsp. poultry seasoning
2 cans Carnation Skim Milk
6 buttermilk biscuits (see recipe)
1 pan cornbread (see recipe)
salt, black pepper, & red pepper to taste

Boil chicken with chicken soup mix until tender. Set aside, reserving at least 4-5 cups of the water. Chop up meat into very small pieces. Soak bread in milk, set aside. Sauté vegetables in oil in heavy pot about 6 minutes, or until tender.

In large pan, mix cornbread, biscuits, vegetable mixture, milk & bread mixture, poultry seasonings, sliced boiled eggs, and chopped chicken breasts with reserved water. Season to taste. Mix together well. Mixture should be very moist. Bake in deep baking dish at 350 degrees for 1 hour or until firm and brown.

Yield .... 24 servings
Serving Size .... ½ cup
Calories 157
Protein 8
Carbs. 13
Fat 7

Breads

CORNBREAD

1 cup corn meal
½ cup whole wheat flour
½ tsp. baking soda
2 tsp. baking powder
½ tsp. salt
1 egg
1 Tbsp. olive oil
1 cup low-fat buttermilk
¼ cup fruit sweetener

Mix dry ingredients together. In blender, mix egg, oil, buttermilk, and sweetener. Pour into flour mixture, mixing well.

Pour into 9" baking dish sprayed with Pam. Bake 25 minutes at 350 degrees or until golden brown.

Yield .... 8 slices
Calories 165
Protein 3
Carbs. 18
Fat 4

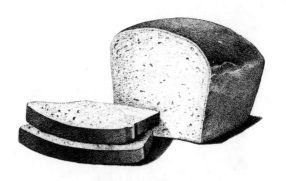

POPOVERS

1 cup whole wheat flour
¼ tsp. salt
3 eggs
1 Tbsp. melted butter
1 cup nonfat milk
2 Tbsp. butter, cut into six small pieces

Preheat oven to 425 degrees. Spray popover pan with Pam and place in middle of preheated oven for about 2 minutes. Blend ingredients together at high speed on mixer or food processor for about 4 minutes. Batter should be very smooth. Place small pieces of butter in popover pan, return to oven about 1 minute until butter is melted. Fill each cup half full with batter. Bake at 400 degrees for 20 minutes, then lower heat to 350 degrees for 30 to 40 minutes or until popovers are done.

```
Yield  . . . . . . . . . . . . . .   Serves 6
Calories  . . . . . . . . . .71
Protein . . . . . . . . . . . .5
Carbs.  . . . . . . . . . . .16
Fat  . . . . . . . . . . . . . . .5
```

BANANA NUT BREAD OR MUFFINS

2 cups overripe bananas
2 eggs
¼ cup olive oil
½ cup water
10 chopped dates
1 Tbsp. vanilla (no sugar kind)
2 cups whole wheat pastry flour
2 Tbsp. Premium Protein Powder (from Neo-Life Co.)
2 tsp. baking powder
½ tsp. baking soda
¼ tsp. salt
½ cup low-fat buttermilk
½ cup chopped walnuts (lightly roasted)

In blender combine bananas, dates, eggs, and vanilla. Gradually add oil, blend well. Sift dry ingredients together in large mixing bowl. With electric mixer alternate dry ingredients and buttermilk to banana combination, mixing well. Fold in nuts.

For bread, pour batter into a 8½" X 4½" greased loaf pan. Bake at 350 degrees for 30 minutes, then reduce heat to 300 degrees and bake until dark brown or until cake test is done. About 30 to 35 minutes.

For muffins, spoon batter into 12 greased muffin cups, filling about ¾ full. Bake at 300 degrees until dark brown, about 1 hour, or until toothpick test comes out clean.

```
Yield .............    Serves 12
Calories ........ 198
Protein .......... 7
Carbs. .......... 24
Fat .............. 9
```

BUCKWHEAT PANCAKES

1 cup buckwheat flour
1 beaten egg
1 Tbsp. melted butter
2 cups buttermilk
1 tsp. baking powder
½ tsp. baking soda
¼ tsp. salt

Blend dry ingredients together. Add butter, egg, and buttermilk, mixing well. Cook over hot grill until bubbles appear on top, flip over, cook for about 3-4 minutes until done.

Yield 12   5" pancakes
Calories 59
Protein 3
Carbs. 8
Fat 2

BUTTERMILK BISCUITS

1 cup whole wheat pastry flour
2 tsp. baking powder
¼ tsp. baking soda
¼ tsp. salt
2 Tbsp. melted butter
⅓ cup buttermilk

Blend dry ingredients together. Add butter and buttermilk. Mixture should be soft. Turn over onto floured board, knead about three times, cut with biscuit cutter. Bake for 20 minutes at 350 degrees or until golden brown.

Yield .... Serves 6
Calories 106
Protein 3
Carbs. 15
Fat 4

SOURDOUGH STARTER

2 packages active dry yeast
2 cups warm water
2 cups whole wheat flour

Dissolve yeast in water in large bowl. Let stand until bubbly, about 10 minutes. Stir in flour, cover tightly and let stand at room temperature for three days. Stir well once per day. After 3 days mix:

Sourdough Feeder

1 cup whole wheat flour
1 cup lowfat buttermilk

Mix well, store in refrigerator loosely covered. Dough has to breathe, so be sure to have hole in top of cover. Feed at least once a week to keep dough alive and active. Use large bowl because dough grows as it ages. By the end of the week dough will have sour smell to it. The older the dough is, the better it is.

Do not get below 1 cup of starter.

Yield . . . . 1 cup
Calories 233
Protein 11
Carbs. 65
Fat 2

SOURDOUGH BISCUITS

1 cup unbleached flour
2 tsp. baking powder
½ tsp. baking soda
¼ tsp. salt
¼ cup olive oil
1 cup starter

Add dry ingredients to oil and starter. Mix until it forms a ball. Knead 4 or 5 times on floured board. Press dough out with fingers. Use biscuit cutter. Bake 12 to 15 minutes at 400 degrees.

```
Yield  . . . . . . . . . . . . . .    Serves 8
Calories  . . . . . . . . .117
Protein  . . . . . . . . . . . .3
Carbs.   . . . . . . . . . . .19
Fat   . . . . . . . . . . . . . . .2
```

SOURDOUGH PANCAKES

The night before, add to 1 cup sourdough starter:
1 cup unbleached flour
1 cup lowfat buttermilk
Let stand in refrigerator overnight. Add:
1 beaten egg
1 tsp. baking soda
¼ tsp. salt
¼ cup melted butter

Add remaining ingredients to sourdough starter, mix well. Spoon over hot grill, brown and turn over. Top with butter and homemade syrup.

```
Yield  . . . . . . . . . . . . . .   Serves 12
Calories  . . . . . . . . . .61
Protein . . . . . . . . . . . .3
Carbs.  . . . . . . . . . .14
Fat  . . . . . . . . . . . . . . .1
```

DATE-NUT MUFFINS

1½ cups pitted dates (no-sugar kind) — Approx. 15 dates
¾ cup boiling water
¼ cup olive oil
1 egg
1 tsp. vanilla
1 tsp. baking powder
½ tsp. baking soda
1½ cups whole wheat pastry flour
¼ tsp. salt
½ cup chopped walnuts

In mixing bowl, mix boiling water, dates, oil, egg, and vanilla. Mix flour, baking powder, baking soda, and salt. Add to date mix. Beat well, fold in walnuts. Spoon into muffin cups and bake at 375 degrees for 25 minutes.

Yield .... 12 muffins
Calories 148
Protein 4
Carbs. 12
Fat 8

OAT BRAN MUFFINS

¼ cup olive oil
1 egg
⅔ cup nonfat milk
1 tsp. baking powder
¾ cup whole wheat flour
2 Tbsp. oat bran
2 Tbsp. wheat germ
¼ cup fruit sweetener

Mix all ingredients with electric mixer. Spoon into muffin cups. Bake at 350 degrees for 45 minutes.

Yield .... 12 muffins
Calories 87
Protein 3
Carbs. 8
Fat 5

BLUEBERRY BREAD SQUARES

1 cup frozen or fresh blueberries (no sugar kind)
1½ cup whole wheat flour
2½ tsp. baking powder
½ tsp. salt
½ cup uncooked oats
2 eggs
¼ cup olive oil
½ cup fruit juice sweetener
½ cup Sweet Cloud Rice Syrup (from health food store)
1 cup mashed bananas

Mix dry ingredients together, set aside. In blender, mix eggs, oil, sweeteners, and bananas until smooth. Pour into dry ingredients, mixing well with electric mixer. Fold in blueberries. Pour into a 33" X 23" X 5" oblong pan sprayed with Pam. Bake for 30 to 35 minutes at 300 degrees.

Yield .... 32 squares
Calories 81
Protein 2
Carbs. 15
Fat 2

VELVET BREAD OR MUFFINS

1 pkg. dry yeast
1 cup warm water
Mix and let stand for 5 minutes.
Add:
1 tsp. salt
¼ cup Sweet Cloud Rice Syrup
1½ cups whole wheat flour

Beat until very creamy in electric mixer, about 5 minutes.

½ cup melted butter
1 egg
1½ to 2 cups whole wheat flour

In electric mixer beat butter into mixture for about 4 minutes. Add egg and beat for 6 minutes, mixture should look velvety. Add flour and mix well in mixer with dough hook. Cover with wet cheesecloth and let rise in a warm place until doubled in size, about 1½ to 2 hours. Punch down, knead on flour board 4 or 5 times. Make sure mixture remains very soft. Place in greased muffin tins or place in two loaf pans. Let rise in warm place, uncovered, until doubled in size. Bake at 350 degrees for about 20-25 minutes or until toothpick test done.

```
Yield  . . . . . . . . . . . . . .   2 loaves — 12 slices per loaf
Calories . . . . . . . . . . . .   61
Protein . . . . . . . . . . . .   2
Carbs.  . . . . . . . . . . . .   4
Fat  . . . . . . . . . . . . . . .   3
```

FRENCH TOAST

2 eggs
½ cup nonfat milk
1 tsp. cinnamon
1 tsp. vanilla (no sugar kind)
4 slices homemade whole wheat bread or Ezekiel bread

Mix eggs, milk, cinnamon, and vanilla together in blender. Pour into deep bowl. Dip bread into mixture, brown each side in frying pan with a little butter. Top with Real Syrup.

Yield	2 servings — 2 slices each
Calories	231
Protein	2
Carbs.	31
Fat	8

HERBED ENGLISH MUFFIN

4 cups whole wheat flour
1 cup gluten flour
1 cup wheat bran
2 pkgs. active dry yeast
1 tsp. marjoram
½ tsp. thyme leaves
½ tsp. oregano
2½ cups warm water
3 Tbsp. concentrated apple juice
1 tsp. sea salt

Combine water, apple juice, yeast in a large bowl. Let sit until yeast activates. Add herbs and gluten flour. Gradually add whole wheat flour while mixing constantly. Add enough flour so that the mixture is quite gooey and slightly stiff. Cover and let rise for about ½ hour. Sprinkle flour on pastry board and knead dough until stiff. Let rise again for about ½ hour. Knead again 6 or 7 times, shape into balls and place in muffin tins. Let rise until double in size.

Bake in preheated 300 degree oven for about 45 minutes or until done.

```
Yield  . . . . . . . . . . . . . .   4 servings
Calories  . . . . . . . . .580
Protein  . . . . . . . . . .34
Carbs.   . . . . . . . . . .114
Fat  . . . . . . . . . . . . . .3
```

Salads and Dressings

RAW VEGETABLE DIP

1 — 6 oz. Yoplait Plain Low-fat Yogurt
1 pint low-fat cottage cheese
3 Tbsp. minced parsley
3 Tbsp. grated onions
3 Tbsp. dill weed
1 tsp. salt

Mix together in blender. Chill before serving. This can be made several days ahead.

Serving Size . . . . 1 Tbsp.
Calories 18
Protein 1
Carbs. 1
Fat . .less than 1 gram

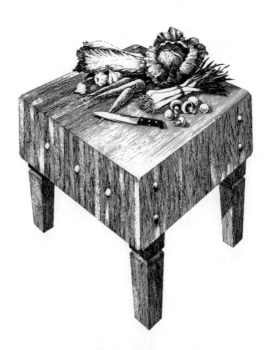

FRESH GUACAMOLE SALAD

1 large avocado
1 small minced onion
1 tsp. salt
1 Tbsp. lemon juice
⅛ tsp. Louisiana Hot Sauce
1 clove minced garlic
2 peeled and chopped tomatoes
1 tsp. chili powder**

**May substitute 2 finely chopped chili peppers instead of chili powder.

Blend together at high speed in mixer or food processor. Serve over a bed of Romaine lettuce or use as a dip.

```
Yield  . . . . . . . . . . . . . .   2 servings
Calories . . . . . . . . .235
Protein . . . . . . . . . . .4
Carbs.  . . . . . . . . . .14
Fat  . . . . . . . . . . . . .19
```

FRUIT SALAD

1 apple
1 orange
1 cup small seedless grapes
2 bananas
1 pear
1 small can unsweetened pineapple chunks (drained)
1 cup chopped dates (no sugar kind)
½ cup chopped walnuts
1 package sugar-free Strawberry Jello
½ pint whipping cream

Cut up fruit in small pieces, add remaining ingredients, mix well. Set aside. In deep mixing bowl, mix whipping cream and Jello gelatin until stiff. Add fruit to whipping cream, mixing well. Serve chilled.

Serving Size . . . .   ½ cup
Calories 62
Protein 1
Carbs. 9
Fat 2

POTATO SALAD

4 medium diced red potatoes
2 boiled eggs
1 Tbsp. minced onions
¼ cup chopped bell pepper
¼ cup chopped celery
¼ cup chopped bread and butter pickles (homemade)
¼ cup chopped olives
½ cup imitation mayonnaise
2 Tbsp. prepared mustard
Salt, pepper, and paprika to taste

Boil potatoes with skins until tender. Drain, add all other ingredients, mix well. Sprinkle with paprika. Serve warm or cold.

Serving Size . . . .   ½ cup
Calories 71
Protein 3
Carbs. 11
Fat 3

FRENCH SALAD

1 head lettuce
1 clove garlic
½ tsp. dry mustard
1 tsp. salt
¼ tsp. pepper
¼ tsp. rice syrup
1 Tbsp. vinegar
2 Tbsp. olive oil
1 Tbsp. chopped parsley

Rub garlic around bowl. Add mustard, salt, pepper, rice syrup, and oil. Blend thoroughly then add the parsley. Wash and dry lettuce leaves and tear gently into pieces. Add to dressing in bowl and toss until thoroughly coated.

Let stand 30 minutes before serving.

```
Yield  . . . . . . . . . . . . .    4 Servings
Calories  . . . . . . . . . .72
Protein . . . . . . . . . . . .0
Carbs.   . . . . . . . . . . .8
Fat  . . . . . . . . . . . . . .7
```

FRUIT AND NUT SALAD

2 cored peeled apples
1 peeled grapefruit, cut into sections
2 cored sliced pears
½ lb. seedless grapes
¾ cup chopped walnuts
½ cup grapefruit juice

Slice apples into wedges and place in bowl with remaining ingredients. Toss and chill. Serve cold. Top with fruit dressing.

```
Yield  .............   Serves 4
Calories  ........312
Protein  ..........6.5
Carbs.  ...........45
Fat  ..............15
```

APPLE STUFFED TOMATOES

4 tomatoes
1 tart diced apple
1 stalk diced celery
1 Tbsp. minced onion
3 Tbsp. real mayonnaise (see recipe)
Chopped olives

Combine ingredients, mix well and chill. Wash and core the tomatoes. Remove insides, drain and chill. Scoop chilled mixture into tomatoes and garnish with chopped olives.

Yield .... Serves 4
Calories 47.5
Protein 1.5
Carbs. 5.5
Fat 6.5

ARTICHOKE SALAD

1 — 14 oz. can artichokes
1 clove minced garlic
½ cup herbed vinaigrette
1 Tbsp. chopped parsley

Drain artichokes and toss with remaining ingredients. Chill. Serve cold.

Yield .... Serves 4
Calories 50
Protein 1.5
Carbs. 9.5
Fat 0

PASTA SALAD

1 cup DeBoles Elbow Macaroni (cooked)
1 lb. boiled shrimp (cleaned and deveined)
1 cup frozen baby early peas
½ cup shredded carrots
¼ cup chopped green onions
¼ cup minced onion
½ cup Remoulade Dressing (see recipe)

Mix all ingredients together. Chill before serving.

Yield	Serves 8
Serving Size	1 cup
Calories 171	
Protein 14	
Carbs. 15	
Fat 12	

CAESAR SALAD

1 head romaine lettuce
1 tsp. dry mustard
½ tsp. salt
¼ tsp. pepper
⅓ cup grated parmesan cheese
6 Tbsp. olive oil
½ squeezed lemon
4 chopped anchovies
1 egg
Croutons

Place egg in boiling water for 3 minutes. Wash, dry, and tear lettuce into bite size pieces. Place lettuce in bowl and sprinkle dry mustard, salt, pepper, and cheese over it. Drip oil over leaves and squeeze lemon juice on top. Add anchovies. Break egg into greens and toss gently, until well coated, but not mushy. Add croutons. Serve immediately.

Yield . . . .   Serves 4
Calories 305.75
Protein 10.5
Carbs. 4
Fat 26¼

GREEN & RAW VEGETABLE SALAD

3 cups Romaine lettuce
½ cup chopped broccoli
½ cup shredded carrots
½ cup chopped cauliflower
¼ cup chopped celery
1 chopped cucumber
1 chopped tomato
1 chopped bell pepper
2 tsp. fresh chives

Mix all ingredients together. Serve with your choice of salad dressing.

```
Serving Size  ........  1
Calories  ..........98
Protein ...........0
Carbs.  ..........21
Fat  ..............0
```

WESTERN SALAD

1 boiled egg
1 head Boston lettuce
½ lb. spinach
1 sliced onion
2 Tbsp. chopped parsley
¼ cup vinegar
½ cup salad oil
1 dash garlic powder
½ tsp. paprika
¼ tsp. dry mustard
1 tsp. salt
¼ tsp. pepper

Remove egg yolk and mash with garlic. Blend in salt, paprika, pepper, and mustard. Add salad oil, vinegar; beat well. Chop egg white and parsley and stir in. Combine lettuce, spinach and onion in salad bowl. Add dressing. Toss lightly.

```
Yield . . . . . . . . . . . . . .   Serves 4
Calories  . . . . . . . . 317
Protein  . . . . . . . . . . 4.3
Carbs. . . . . . . . . . .  10
Fat . . . . . . . . . . . . . .  22
```

SPINACH ALMOND SALAD

10 ozs. fresh spinach
1 cup slivered almonds
1 hard boiled egg
6 Tbsp. olive oil
2 Tbsp. wine vinegar
1 tsp. salt
¼ tsp. pepper

Make dressing with olive oil, wine vinegar, salt and pepper. Wash and dry spinach; tear into bite sized pieces. Place in salad bowl and scatter almonds over it. Toss lightly with dressing and top with chopped egg.

Yield .... Serves 4
Calories 419
Protein 9
Carbs. 8
Fat 22

APPLE VEGETABLE MOLD

1 pkg. plain gelatin
¼ cup hot water
1 cup boiling apple cider
¼ cup white vinegar
2 Tbsp. lemon juice
½ tsp. salt
1 large peeled cucumber
⅓ cup chopped cabbage
2 Tbsp. chopped onion
½ cup chopped celery
1 grated carrot
2 Tbsp. chopped green pepper
1 peeled grated apple

Soak gelatin in hot water for 3 minutes. Add salt. Cut cucumber lengthwise, remove the seeds; chop. Combine ingredients and chill.

```
Yield . . . . . . . . . . . . . .   Serves 4
Calories  . . . . . . . . . 66
Protein  . . . . . . . . . . . 1
Carbs. . . . . . . . . . . 21
Fat . . . . . . . . . . . . . . 0
```

PASTA BEAN SALAD

1 cup steamed green beans
1 cup cooked kidney beans
½ cup sliced black olives
⅓ cup chopped onion
½ cup cooked wheat noodles
⅔ cup olive oil
⅓ cup vinegar
Dash salt & pepper
Dash paprika
½ clove finely minced garlic

Mix cooked beans, olives, onion, and noodles together. In a separate bowl mix oil, vinegar, seasonings and garlic together. Stir dressing well.
Pour over bean mixture and marinate for several hours. Serve chilled.

***NOTE: To turn this hefty salad into a main dish delight, add chunks of steamed chilled white fish or chunks of cooked, cubed chicken to the bean noodle mix before adding the dressing.

Yield . . . .   Serves 4
Calories 283
Protein 5
Carbs. 19
Fat 17

LETTUCE AND BEAN SPROUTS SALAD

1 head Romaine lettuce
3 cups fresh bean sprouts
3 large sliced tomatoes
1 large sliced onion
2 Tbsp. fresh basil
3 cloves garlic
⅓ cup olive oil**
¼ cup wine vinegar
Pinch Cajun seasoning to taste
Sesame seeds

**Use cold pressed olive oil

Toss together all fresh ingredients. Blend dressing and pour over salad. Sprinkle with sesame seeds.

Yield . . . . Serves 4
Calories 97
Protein 3
Carbs. 22
Fat 18

IMITATION MAYONNAISE

1 cup low-fat cottage cheese
1 Tbsp. lemon juice
1 Tbsp. Sweet Cloud Rice Syrup

Mix all ingredients in blender. Store in glass jar in the refrigerator.

Serving Size . . . . 1 Tbsp.
Calories 23
Protein 3
Carbs. 1.5
Fat . . less than 1 gram

REAL MAYONNAISE

1 egg
½ tsp. salt
1 tsp. mustard
3 Tbsp. lemon juice
½ cup olive oil
½ cup safflower oil

Mix egg, salt, mustard, and lemon juice in blender or food processor. Add oil very slowly. Mixture should be very thick. Refrigerate in tightly sealed container.

Yield	2 cups
Serving Size	1 Tbsp.
Calories 65	
Protein 0	
Carbs. 0	
Fat 14	

REMOULADE DRESSING

2 cups Real mayonnaise (see recipe)
3 large garlic pods
3 green onion bottoms
1 Tbsp. chopped parsley
2 tsp. horseradish (no sugar kind)
3 tsp. Creole mustard

Mix all ingredients in blender or food processor until smooth. Store in tightly sealed jar in refrigerator.

```
Yield  .............. 3 cups
Serving Size ........ 1 Tbsp.
Calories ..........68
Protein ............0
Carbs.  ............3
Fat  ..............14
```

ITALIAN DRESSING

1 cup olive oil
¼ tsp. salt
¼ tsp. onion powder
¼ tsp. dried minced onions
¼ tsp. oregano
¼ tsp. garlic powder
¼ tsp. pepper
¼ cup cider vinegar
1 Tbsp. lemon juice
1 tsp. rice syrup
1 Tbsp. water

Blend all ingredients in blender or food processor until well mixed.

Serving Size . . . .   1 Tbsp.
Calories 90
Protein 0
Carbs. 0
Fat 11

DIET DRESSING

¼ cup boiling water
2 tsp. plain gelatin
¾ cup cold water
1 Tbsp. honey
1 tsp. dry mustard
¼ tsp. salt
1 Tbsp. olive oil
1 clove minced garlic
¼ cup vinegar

In a sauce pan dissolve gelatin in hot water. Add cold water, honey, mustard, and salt. Heat and cook 5 minutes. Add oil and garlic. Cook until thickened. Remove from heat; stir in vinegar and chill. Shake before serving.

```
Yield  .............  Serves 4
Calories  .........47
Protein ............0
Carbs.  ............4
Fat  ..............4
```

FRUIT DRESSING

½ cup fresh buttermilk
½ cup real mayonnaise
1 Tbsp. Rice Syrup
1 Tbsp. fresh lemon juice
1 tsp. grated lemon rind

In medium size bowl, mix buttermilk, rice syrup, lemon juice, and lemon rind. Fold in mayonnaise. Serve over fruit or sweet vegetables.

Yield . . . . Serves 4
Calories 46
Protein 2
Carbs. 7
Fat 2

Mini-Meals

VEGETARIAN PROTEIN DRINK

1 cup pineapple juice (no sugar kind)
1 cup water
1 frozen banana
2 Tbsp. vegetarian protein powder

   Mix all ingredients in blender until well blended.

   Serving Size ....   6 oz.
   Calories 56
   Protein 4
   Carbs. 10
   Fat 0

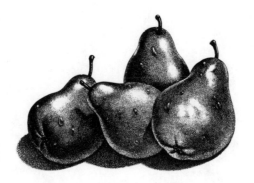

PEANUT BUTTER D'LIGHT

1 box whole grain cereal (no sugar kind)
½ cup olive oil
1 pint crunchy peanut butter (no sugar kind)
1 cup lightly roasted pecans
¼ cup cold water

Process cereal in blender or food processor until powdered. Mix cereal, peanut butter, olive oil, and water together with a fork. Add pecans, mix well. Set in refrigerator for about 2 hours to harden. After mixture has set, roll into balls and place on wax paper. Return to refrigerator while you make Carob Dip (see following recipe).

CAROB DIP

1 cup water
2 cups unsweetened carob chips
1 inch paraffin wax
1 tsp. vanilla (no sugar kind)
¼ cup Rice Syrup
1 Tbsp. butter

Bring water and paraffin to boil. Lower heat, add carob chips, and rice syrup stirring constantly so carob doesn't burn. When mixture is dark and creamy, remove from heat. Add vanilla and butter. Mix well.

Dip peanut butter balls into carob dip mixture using tongs and place on wax paper. Return to refrigerator for approximately 3 hours to set.

Store in sealed bowl or Ziploc bag when completely hardened.

Yield .... 48 balls
Calories 130
Protein 3
Carbs. 23
Fat 9

GRANOLA

1½ cups uncooked oats
1 cup fresh coconut (no sugar kind)
¼ cup pumpkin seeds
1 cup sunflower seeds
½ cup wheat germ

Mix well then add:

½ cup Sweet Cloud Rice Syrup
½ cup ice water
¼ cup olive oil

Mix well, spread in deep oblong baking dish sprayed with Pam. Bake at 225 degrees for 1½ hours. Add:

1 cup chopped pecans
1 cup chopped walnuts
1 cup chopped almonds
Mix, continue to bake ½ hour longer. Add:
½ cup raisins
½ cup chopped dates (no sugar kind)

Mix well, let cool and store in Ziploc bags.

Yield . . . .   Approx. 10 cups
Serving Size . . . .   1 Tbsp.
Calories 53
Protein 2
Carbs. 4
Fat 3

CAROB MINT CUPS

½ cup water
1 cup unsweetened carob chips
1 tsp. vanilla (no sugar kind)
2 tsp. butter
¼ cup Rice Syrup
Approx. ½ inch square paraffin wax
12 foil muffin cups

In heavy pot bring water and paraffin wax to boil. Lower heat. Add carob chips, and rice syrup stirring constantly until smooth and creamy. Remove from heat. Add vanilla and butter. Mix well. Spray foil cups with Pam before filling. Fill foil muffin cups about ⅓ full of mixture. Put aside to set. Prepare mint filling as follows.

MINT FILLING

1 pkg. Light Neufchatel Cream Cheese
1 cup low-fat cottage cheese
½ tsp. peppermint extract (no sugar kind)
1 tsp. vanilla (no sugar kind)
1 Tbsp. warm water
¼ cup Rice Syrup
½ cup chopped nuts

In blender or food processor, mix cream cheese, cottage cheese, and rice syrup until smooth. Add the vanilla and peppermint flavorings. Blend into cream cheese mixture. Place in refrigerator about 30 minutes to set. Fill carob cups with approximately 3 tablespoons of filling. Top with chopped nuts. Chill in refrigerator 2 hours or until set before serving.

Yield .... 12 muffin cups
Calories 179
Protein 5
Carbs. 8
Fat 14

Desserts

BUTTER/NUT PIE CRUST

1½ cup whole wheat flour
¼ cup finely ground walnuts
¼ tsp. salt
⅓ cup olive oil
¼ cup buttermilk
¼ cup cold water

    Combine dry ingredients. Add oil, buttermilk, and water. Mix well with a fork. Pat out into a 9" pie shell. Bake at for 20 minutes at 350° or until golden brown for recipes calling for cooked shell.

      Yield .... 2 pie shells
      Serving Size .... 8 slices per pie
      Calories 77
      Protein 2
      Carbs. 8
      Fat 4

BUTTERMILK PIE CRUST

1 cup whole wheat pastry flour
½ cup softened butter
¼ tsp. salt
3 Tbsp. buttermilk

Blend flour, butter, and salt together with pastry cutter. Add buttermilk, mix with fork. Roll out on floured board or waxed paper. Press out into a 9" pie plate. Bake at 350 degrees for 25 minutes.

Yield .... 8 slices
Calories 79
Protein 2
Carbs. 11
Fat 3

BANANA CREAM PIE

1 cup plain nonfat yogurt
1 cup low-fat cottage cheese
1 package sugar free instant vanilla pudding
1 tsp. vanilla (no sugar kind)
2 bananas
1 envelope Knox Gelatin
2 Tbsp. warm water
2 Tbsp. rice syrup
1 butter/nut pie crust

Dissolve gelatin in warm water, set aside. In blender or food processor, mix yogurt, cottage cheese, rice syrup, and vanilla until smooth. Add banana and gelatin mixture, blend until smooth. Place in cooled cooked butter/nut pie crust.

Place in refrigerator until set, about 2 hours.

```
Yield  .............. 8 slices
Calories  .........160
Protein .............7
Carbs.  ...........23
Fat  ..............4
```

PECAN PIE

1 egg
4 egg whites
¼ tsp. salt
1 15-oz. jar Sweet Cloud Rice Syrup
¼ cup fruit sweetener
2 tsp. vanilla (no sugar kind)
2 cups pecans (lightly roasted)
2 uncooked buttermilk pie crust

Combine all ingredients (except pecans) in blender or food processor, mixing well. Place 1 cup pecans in each uncooked pie shell. Pour ½ of mixture into each shell and bake at 300 degrees for 1 hour.

Yield — 2 pies — 8 slices each

Serving Size	1 slice
Calories 203	
Protein 25	
Carbs. 27	
Fat 9	

Total Cal. w/Pie Crust:

Calories 280	
Protein 4	
Carbs. 35	
Fat 13	

YOGURT CHERRY PIE

1 — 16 oz. tub of plain nonfat yogurt
½ pint whipping cream
1 Tbsp. warm water
1 pkg. unflavored gelatin
1 tsp. vanilla (no sugar kind)
3 Tbsp. Sweet Cloud Rice Syrup
1 cup fresh pitted and sliced cherries

Dissolve gelatin in warm water. Add to whipping cream with syrup and vanilla. Whip until stiff. Fold in yogurt and cherries. Pour into a 9" cooked and cooled Butter/Nut Pie Crust. Place in freezer about 4 hours. Remove from freezer for approximately 30 minutes before serving.

Yield .... 8 slices
Calories .... .242
Protein 6
Carbs. 24
Fat 13

STRAWBERRY PIE

1 pint fresh strawberries
1 envelope Knox unflavored gelatin
¾ cup water
2 egg whites
¼ tsp. cream of tartar
1 Tbsp. lemon juice
2 Tbsp. Westbrae Natural Strawberry Conserves
½ cup whipped whipping cream
1 cooked 9" Butter/Nut Pie Crust

Crush strawberries, set aside. In a heavy pot, heat water, gelatin, lemon juice, and strawberry conserves until well dissolved. Add crushed strawberries, mix well. Chill until mixture mounds when spooned. Fold in whipped cream.

Beat egg whites with cream of tartar until soft peaks form. Fold into strawberry mixture. Pour into 9" pie crust. Chill about 1 hour to set. Top with extra whipped cream and whole strawberries.

```
Yield  . . . . . . . . . . . . .  8 slices
Calories  . . . . . . . .194
Protein . . . . . . . . . . .4
Carbs.  . . . . . . . . . .12
Fat  . . . . . . . . . . . . .14
```

BLUEBERRIES SUPREME

Filling

2 — 8 oz. softened Philadelphia Light Cream Cheese
1 tsp. vanilla (no sugar kind)
½ cup Sweet Cloud Rice Syrup
1 egg

Process in blender or food processor until smooth. Set aside.

½ pint whipping cream
1 tsp. vanilla
1 cooked Butter/Nut Pie Crust pressed into a 9" X 13" baking pan

In mixing bowl, mix all ingredients until stiff. Add cream cheese mixture and blend with spatula. Spread over cooled crust. Set in refrigerator about 1 hour to set.

Topping

1 pint fresh blueberries, washed and drained
1 cup water
1 Tbsp. whole wheat flour
½ tsp. cinnamon
1 tsp. vanilla (no sugar kind)
½ cup fruit sweetener

Bring water and flour to boil, add cinnamon and fruit sweetener. Add berries and mix well, cook about 10 minutes until mixture is thick. Remove from heat. Add vanilla, mix well. Place in refrigerator about 1 hour or until mixture has completely cooled. Pour over pie filling. Let set about 1 hour until firm. Fresh strawberries or other fresh fruits may be substituted with excellent results.

Yield .... 12 — 1½" X 2" pieces

Total Calories-Supreme & Topping	Topping Calories:
Calories 179	Calories 46
Protein 3	Protein ....trace
Carbs. 19	Carbs. 12
Fat 11	Fat ....trace

FRESH PEAR PIE

3 cups diced and cored raw pears, approx. 4 pears
1 tsp. cinnamon
1 Tbsp. whole wheat flour
½ cup Sweet Cloud Rice Syrup
1 Tbsp. butter
1 uncooked Butter/Nut Pie Crust

Mix pears, cinnamon, flour, and rice syrup together. Pour into pie shell, dot with butter. Cover with strips of remaining pie crust. Bake at 425 degrees for 40 to 45 minutes. Pears will be crunchy.

```
Yield ..............    8 slices
Calories ........ 196
Protein .......... 3
Carbs. .......... 35
Fat .............. 6
```

CHERRY PIE

3 cups fresh pitted cherries
½ cup water
1 Tbsp. whole wheat flour
1 tsp. vanilla (no sugar kind)
½ tsp. cinnamon
½ cup Sweet Cloud Rice Syrup
Whipped Cream Topping (see recipe)
1 cooked 9" buttermilk pie crust

Combine cherries, water, cinnamon, flour, and rice syrup. Cook over medium heat until thick. Remove from heat. Add vanilla and mix well. Spoon into cooked pie shell. Cool for 1 hour. Top with Whipped Cream Topping.

Yield .... 8 slices
Calories 204
Protein 4
Carbs. 22
Fat 12

CHOCOLATE CREAM PIE

2 cups nonfat milk
1 egg yolk
1 Tbsp. whole wheat flour
1 tsp. vanilla
1 tsp. chocolate extract (no sugar kind)
3 Tbsp. carob powder (no sugar kind)
½ cup Sweet Cloud Rice Syrup
Whip Cream Topping
1 cooked buttermilk pie shell

In heavy pot, cook milk, egg yolk, flour, and carob powder over medium heat until thick. Remove from fire. Add vanilla, chocolate extract, and rice syrup. Mixture will thicken more as it cools. Place in cooled pie shell. Let cool for 1 hour to set. Top with Whip Cream Topping.

Yield . . . . .8 slices	Total Calories of Whole Pie	
Calories — Pie alone 212	Cal. — Pie with Whip Cream .700	
Protein 5	Protein 5	
Carbs. 19	Carbs. 7	
Fat 13	Fat 74	

DEVAN APPLE PIE

6 baking apples (peeled and diced)
1 tsp. cinnamon
¼ tsp. cloves
¼ tsp. nutmeg
¼ tsp. salt
3 Tbsp. cornstarch
3 Tbsp. whole wheat flour
2 cups Devan Sweet
1 Tbsp. butter (cut in four squares)
1 egg beaten
2 uncooked buttermilk pie crusts
(2 uncooked buttermilk pie crusts for topping pies)

Core and peel apples, dice into bowl of lightly salted water, set aside.

Combine: cinnamon, spices, cornstarch, flour and Devan Sweet, mix well. Drain apples, fold into dry ingredients, making sure apples are well coated.

Pour mixture into two uncooked pie shells; dot with two squares of butter each. Top each pie with other pie crust. Brush both pies with beaten egg, sprinkle each pie evenly with one tablespoon of Devan Sweet. Cut several slits in top of each pie with sharp knife. Bake at 350 degrees for 45 minutes.

Yield .... 2 pies, 8 slices each
Calories 231.5
Protein 2
Carbs. 34
Fat 4.5

PUMPKIN PIE

1 — 16 oz. can pumpkin (no sugar kind)
1 cup nonfat milk
1 tsp. ground cinnamon
½ tsp. ground nutmeg
¼ tsp. ground ginger
¼ tsp. ground cloves
¼ tsp. salt
3 eggs
¼ tsp. cream of tartar
½ cup fruit sweetener
1 uncooked buttermilk pie shell

Combine pumpkin, milk, and spices. Mix well. Separate 1 egg, set white aside. Combine yolk and remaining 2 eggs, mixing well. Add to pumpkin mixture, add sweetener and mix well. Beat egg white with cream of tartar until stiff. Fold into pumpkin mixture. Pour into unbaked pie shell. Bake at 425 degrees for 45 minutes or until firm in center.

Yield .... 8 slices
Calories 182
Protein 6
Carbs. 24
Fat 7

SWEET POTATO PIE

4 medium sweet potatoes
1 cup evaporated skim milk
2 eggs
1 tsp. ground cinnamon
½ tsp. ground nutmeg
¼ tsp. ground ginger
⅛ tsp. ground cloves
¼ tsp. salt
½ cup fruit sweetener
¼ cup raisins
½ cup chopped walnuts
1 uncooked buttermilk pie crust

Bake sweet potatoes until tender, about 1¾ hours. Peel potatoes, and place in deep mixing bowl. Combine milk, eggs, fruit sweetener, and spices, and mix well with electric mixer. Fold in nuts and raisins. Bake at 400 degrees for 45 minutes or until center is firm.

Pie may be topped with Whip Cream Topping if desired.

Yield .... 8 slices

Calories without Whip Cream Topping
Calories 294
Protein 7
Carbs. 43
Fat 11

BLACKBERRY COBBLER

1 pint washed and drained fresh blackberries
1 cup water
1 Tbsp. whole wheat flour
½ tsp. cinnamon
1 tsp. vanilla
½ cup rice syrup
2 uncooked buttermilk pie crusts, 1 whole and 1 cut into strips

Bring water and flour to boil. Add berries, cinnamon, vanilla, and rice syrup. Cook until thick, about 10 minutes. In deep, oblong, baking dish, press in pie dough. Add ½ of berries, cover with strips of dough, pour in rest of mixture and top with remaining strips of pie dough. Bake at 350 degrees for 30 to 40 minutes or until golden brown.

Yield	Approx. 12 — 1½" pieces
Calories	163
Protein	3
Carbs.	25
Fat	6

STRAWBERRY LITE PIE

1 cup plain nonfat yogurt
1 — 8 oz. pkg. Light Philadelphia Neufchatel Cream Cheese
1 package sugar free instant vanilla pudding
2 cups fresh strawberries
1 pkg. Sugar Free Strawberry Jello
1 tsp. vanilla
½ cup fruit sweetener
1 cup water
1 cooked and cooled Butter/Nut pie shell

In blender, mix vanilla, instant vanilla pudding, yogurt, and cream cheese until smooth. Set aside. Wash strawberries, drain, and cut up into slices. Set aside. In heavy pot, bring water, and fruit sweetener to boil, add Jello and mix well. Cool in refrigerator until lightly set. Add strawberries and mix well.

Fill cooked pie shell with cheese mixture and top with strawberry mixture. Cool 1 hour before serving.

```
Yield  . . . . . . . . . . . . . .   Serves 8
Calories  . . . . . . . . .203
Protein  . . . . . . . . . . .6
Carbs.   . . . . . . . . . .27
Fat  . . . . . . . . . . . . .11
```

CARROT CAKE

2 cups whole wheat pastry flour
1 Tbsp. baking powder
½ tsp. baking soda
½ tsp. salt
2 tsp. cinnamon
½ tsp. nutmeg
½ cup olive oil
1 cup pitted dates, approx. 10 dates
½ cup buttermilk
4 eggs
2½ cups grated carrots
1 — 8 oz. can crushed unsweetened pineapple
1 cup chopped & roasted walnuts
½ cup raisins
1 Tbsp. vanilla (no sugar kind)

Sift flour, baking powder, soda, salt, cinnamon, and nutmeg together. In blender, combine olive oil, dates, eggs, buttermilk, and vanilla, blend well. In large mixing bowl, combine flour mixture with grated carrots. Slowly add mixture from blender, mixing well after each addition. Add crushed pineapple, mix well. Stir in raisins and walnuts. Place mixture into well greased and floured 9" X 13" baking pan. Bake at 350 degrees for 40-45 minutes or until cake tests done. Cool completely. Top with Sour Cream Frosting.

```
Yield .............   24 slices
Calories  ........ 140
Protein  .......... 4
Carbs. ...........  15
Fat ...............  8
```

BIRTHDAY CAKE

2½ cups Unbleached white flour
2½ tsp. baking powder
½ tsp. baking soda
½ tsp. salt
3 eggs
2 sticks softened butter
1 — 15 oz. jar Sweet Cloud Rice Syrup
½ cup organic fruit sweetener
1 Tbsp. vanilla flavoring (no sugar kind)
2 tsp. coconut flavoring (no sugar kind)
1 cup low-fat buttermilk

Sift together dry ingredients, set aside. With an electric mixer, beat butter and rice syrup together until creamy.

Add eggs, one at a time, beating well after each addition. Add fruit sweetener, flavorings, and buttermilk, mixing well. Slowly add flour mixture, beating well after each addition. Beat at least 3 minutes after the last amount of flour has been added. Pour into two 9" round cake pans, sprayed generously with Pam. Bake 45 minutes at 350 degrees, until cake tests done. Cool well before topping with filling. Top with top layer and frost.

Yield .... 27 — 1" slices

Calories for cake alone:
Calories 161
Protein 3
Carbs. 21
Fat 8

CUSTARD FILLING

1 cup nonfat milk
2 egg yolks
1½ Tbsp. unbleached white flour
¼ tsp. salt
½ tsp. vanilla flavoring
½ tsp. coconut flavoring
¼ cup Sweet Cloud Rice Syrup

In heavy pot, cook milk, yolks, flour, and salt over medium heat until slightly thick. Remove from heat. Add flavorings and rice syrup, mix well. Place in refrigerator for 1 hour. Mixture will thicken as it cools. Pour over cooled cake layer, top with other layer.

Yield . . . . 1½ cups

Calories for pudding only:
Calories 204
Protein 12
Carbs. 26
Fat 7

EIGHT MINUTE COCONUT FROSTING

2 unbeaten egg whites
1 cup Sweet Cloud Rice Syrup
¼ tsp. cream of tartar
⅓ cup water
¼ tsp. salt
1 Tbsp. vanilla flavoring
2 tsp. coconut flavoring

Place egg whites, rice syrup, cream of tartar, water and salt in top of double boiler. Beat constantly with electric mixer until frosting forms peaks, about 6 minutes. Remove from heat. Pour into mixing bowl. Add flavorings. Beat at high speed until mixture is of spreading consistency, about 8 minutes.

Yield .... 5 cups

Calories for frosting only
Calories 719
Protein 6
Carbs. 185
Fat 0

Yield .... 27 — 1" slices

Total Calories for Cake, Filling, & Frosting — 1 slice
Calories 195
Protein 4
Carbs. 29
Fat 8

STRAWBERRY SHORT CAKE

1 recipe Birthday Cake (see Recipe)
1 bottle strawberry syrup (R.W. Knudsen-Pourable Strawberry Topping)
1 pint fresh or frozen strawberries (if frozen is used, use no sugar added brand)

In blender, blend strawberries and syrup for a few seconds. Pour over warm cake layer, top with top layer, pour over remaining strawberry mixture over cake. Place in refrigerator to cool several hours. Top with whip cream (optional).

```
Yield  . . . . . . . . . . . . . .   27 — 1 inch slices
Calories  . . . . . . . . .189
Protein . . . . . . . . . . . .3
Carbs.  . . . . . . . . . . .28
Fat  . . . . . . . . . . . . . .8
```

CAROB CHIP PROTEIN CAKE

1½ cups whole wheat flour
1½ cups unbleached flour
¼ cup Premium Protein Powder (Neo-Life Co. Brand)
½ tsp. baking soda
2 tsp. baking powder
1 tsp. salt
3 eggs
⅔ cup olive oil
1 Tbsp. vanilla
1 cup rice syrup
10 pitted dates
1¼ cups buttermilk
1 cup chopped pecans
1 cup unsweetened carob chips

Sift dry ingredients together, set aside. In blender,mix eggs, oil, vanilla, rice syrup, and dates until smooth. Pour into large mixing bowl, slowly adding dry ingredients, alternating with buttermilk, until well mixed. Fold in nuts and carob chips. Pour into greased 9" Bundt cake pan. Bake at 350 degrees for 45-50 minutes or until cake tests done.

Yield .... 24 — 1" slices
Calories 213
Protein 12
Carbs. 36
Fat 9

NO SUGAR ALMOND ORANGE CAKE

1 — 2½ oz. pkg. slivered almonds
½ cup butter
½ cup olive oil
10 chopped dates (no sugar kind)
3 eggs, separated
2 Tbsp. orange juice
1 tsp. grated orange rind
1 tsp. grated lemon rind
1 Tbsp. vanilla extract
2 tsp. almond extract
1½ cups whole wheat pastry flour
1 cup unbleached white pastry flour
4 tsp. baking powder
½ tsp. baking soda
¾ tsp. sea salt
4 Tbsp. buttermilk powder (Saco brand)
¾ cup water
½ tsp. cream of tartar

Cream butter and olive oil. add egg yolks, beat well. Add lemon rind, orange rind, orange juice and extracts, beat well. Add dates, beat well. Combine flours, baking powder, soda, salt, and buttermilk powder. Mix well. Add dry ingredients to creamed mixture alternately with water. Set batter aside. Beat egg whites (at room temperature) with cream of tartar until stiff peaks form. Fold egg white mixture into reserved batter, add almonds, continue to fold in slowly. Pour batter into well greased 9" Bundt pan. Bake at 350 degrees for 1 hour or until cake tests done. When cake has cooled, pour glaze over top. (See glaze recipe next.)

Yield .... 24 — 1" slices (without glaze)
Calories 151
Protein 3
Carbs. 16
Fat 6

GLAZE

½ cup orange juice
½ jar orange marmalade (Sorrel Ridge Brand from health food store)
1 pkg. Knox unflavored gelatin

Mix orange juice with marmalade and gelatin. Heat until well dissolved. Remove from heat. Mix well. Cool until slightly thick. Spoon over cooled cake.

Glaze only

Yield .... 1 cup
Calories 120
Protein 2
Carbs. 28
Fat 0

Cake with glaze

Yield ..24 — 1" slices
Calories 116
Protein 3
Carbs. 17
Fat 6

CARDAMON WALNUT CAKE

½ cup softened butter
3 eggs
1 Tbsp. grated orange rind
1 Tbsp. grated lemon rind
3 Tbsp. Saco buttermilk powder
1½ cups whole wheat pastry flour
1 cup unbleached white pastry flour
1 Tbsp. baking powder
1 tsp. ground cardamom
2 tsp. vanilla extract
½ cup water
10 chopped dates (no sugar kind)
¾ cup chopped walnuts

In mixing bowl, combine butter, eggs, orange rinds,lemon rinds, and vanilla. Beat until smooth. Add dates, beat until smooth. In another bowl combine flours, baking powder, cardamom and buttermilk powder. Add alternately with water to the egg mixture. Beat well. Fold in walnuts. Pour into well greased 9" Bundt pan. Bake at 350 degrees for 45 minutes or until cake tests done.

Yield . . . . 24 — 1" slices
Calories 123
Protein 4
Carbs. 16
Fat 7

COCONUT-BLACK WALNUT CAKE

1 cup oil
4 eggs
1 cup buttermilk
1½ cups whole wheat pastry flour
1½ cups unbleached white flour
½ tsp. salt
1 tsp. baking soda
1 Tbsp. baking powder
2 tsp. vanilla extract
2 tsp. coconut extract
½ cup fruit sweetener
½ cup chopped black walnuts
1 cup fresh toasted coconut
Coconut Syrup (see recipe)

Combine oil, eggs, sweetener, and extracts; beat well. Combine dry ingredients and add to egg mixture alternately with buttermilk. Beat well after each addition. Fold in nuts and coconut. Pour into Bundt pan sprayed with Pam. Bake at 325 degrees for 1 hour and 5 minutes, or until cake tests done. Pour hot coconut syrup over hot cake. Allow cake to remain in pan for 1 hour. Turn cake out on serving dish. Garnish with ½ cup toasted coconut.

Yield .... 24 slices
Calories 175
Protein 4
Carbs. 16
Fat 12

COCONUT SYRUP

½ cup water
¼ cup butter
1 envelope Knox gelatin
1 tsp. coconut extract (no sugar kind)
¼ cup Sweet Cloud Rice Syrup

Combine gelatin, water, and butter, bring to a boil. Remove from heat, stir in extract and rice syrup. Pour over cake while it is still hot in pan.

Syrup Calories

Calories 5
Protein . . . . .trace
Carbs. 1
Fat 1

Cake & Syrup Calories

Calories 184
Protein 4
Carbs. 16
Fat 13

SOUR CREAM ICING

1 cup low-fat sour cream
1 tsp. vanilla extract
¼ cup Sweet Cloud Rice Syrup

Mix together in mixing bowl. Cool in refrigerator for 1 hour. Spoon over cooled cake.

```
Yield  . . . . . . . . . . . . . .  1½ cups
Calories . . . . . . . . .338
Protein . . . . . . . . . . .15
Carbs.  . . . . . . . . . . . .8
Fat  . . . . . . . . . . . . . .23
```

EIGHT MINUTE FROSTING

2 unbeaten egg whites
1 cup Sweet Cloud Rice Syrup
¼ tsp. cream of tartar
⅓ cup water
¼ tsp. salt
2 tsp. vanilla

Place all ingredients except vanilla in top of double boiler. Beat constantly with electric mixer until frosting forms peaks, about 6 minutes. Remove from heat. Pour into mixing bowl, add vanilla. Beat at high speed until mixture is of spreading consistency, about 6 to 8 minutes.

Calories 719
Protein 6
Carbs. 185
Fat 0

CAROB MINT CHEESECAKE

Filling

1½ cups low-fat cottage cheese
¼ cup carob powder
2 eggs
1 tsp. vanilla extract
¼ tsp. peppermint extract
3 Tbsp. Sweet Cloud Rice Syrup

Mix all ingredients in blender. Pour into a 9" coconut crust pie shell. Bake at 375 degrees for 30-35 minutes.

Calories 103
Protein 8
Carbs. 12
Fat 2

COCONUT CRUST

½ cup chopped walnuts
¼ cup fresh shredded coconut
2 Tbsp. wheat germ
1 Tbsp. melted butter

Mix all ingredients well. Pat mixture over a 9" pie plate.

Calories 76
Protein 2
Carbs. 2
Fat 7

Topping

¼ cup shredded toasted coconut
½ cup chopped walnuts

Sprinkle over top of pie after it has cooled.

Calories 57
Protein 1
Carbs. 1
Fat 5

Yield . . . .   8 slices
Total Calories 236
Total Protein 11
Total Carbs. 15
Total Fat 14

APPLE CINNAMON STRUDEL

1 cup whole wheat flour
1 tsp. baking powder
¼ tsp. baking soda
1 beaten egg
2 Tbsp. olive oil
½ cup apple juice (no sugar kind)
1 tsp. vanilla
1 tsp. cinnamon
1 Tbsp. raisins
½ cup jelly or jam (no sugar kind)
¼ cup chopped walnuts

Glaze

½ tsp. cinnamon
¼ cup Sweet Cloud Rice Syrup
1 Tbsp. melted butter

Mix dry ingredients together. Add egg, olive oil, apple juice, and vanilla. Mix well with electric mixer. Spread dough out onto floured board or wax paper. Knead dough lightly; roll out into rectangular shape approximately 8" X 10". Spread with jam, sprinkle with cinnamon, raisins, and nuts. Roll lengthwise. Place seam-side down onto a cookie sheet sprayed with Pam. Bake 23-30 minutes at 350 degrees. When done, brush top with mixture of cinnamon, rice syrup, and melted butter. Serve warm.

Yield .... 12 slices
Calories 129
Protein 2
Carbs. 14
Fat 3

COCONUT DATE SQUARES

½ cup butter (1 stick)
½ cup Sweet Cloud Rice Syrup
1¼ cup whole wheat flour
2¼ cup fresh coconut
2 eggs
1 tsp. vanilla
1 cup chopped dates (approx. 10 large)
1 tsp. baking powder
¼ cup chopped walnuts
¼ cup raisins

PART 1:

With electric mixer, beat butter with rice syrup until smooth and light. By hand: stir in 1 cup flour and 1 cup coconut. Press into 9" square pan, lightly sprayed with Pam. Bake at 350 degrees for 15 minutes or until golden brown. Remove from oven and set aside.

PART 2:

With electric mixer, beat eggs and vanilla, add dates and beat well. By hand stir in: ¼ cup flour, add baking powder. Add raisins, 1 cup coconut, and walnuts. Mix well with fork. Pour over crust in pan. Bake 10-15 minutes or until golden brown. Remove from oven.

Cool, then garnish with ¼ cup coconut.

Yield .... 25 squares
Calories 125
Protein 3
Carbs. 15
Fat 7

APPLESAUCE BREAD PUDDING

2½ cups nonfat dry milk
2 eggs
8 slices Applesauce Bread or Homemade Whole Wheat Bread
1 cup fruit sweetener
2 tsp. vanilla
1½ tsp. cinnamon
¼ tsp. salt
½ cup seedless raisins
½ cup chopped walnuts

In blender combine milk, eggs and sweetener. Blend until smooth. Add vanilla, cinnamon and salt. Blend well. Break bread slices into small pieces; place into an 8" round baking dish. Pour mixture over bread making sure that bread is well soaked. Top with raisins and walnuts.

Bake at 350 degrees for 40-45 minutes. Mixture should be a little moist.

Yield .... 15 – ½ cup servings
Calories 142
Protein 4
Carbs. 30
Fat 4

PECAN TARTS

Cream Cheese Crust

1 — 3 oz. pkg. softened Philadelphia Light Cream Cheese
½ cup softened butter
1 cup whole wheat flour

Mix together cream cheese and butter in electric mixer. Add flour and mix. Roll into balls about 1" thick. Form into tart pans with fingers.

Filling

½ cup melted butter
¼ tsp. salt
1 egg
4 egg whites
1 15-oz. jar Sweet Cloud Rice Syrup
1 cup pecans (lightly roasted)

Mix in blender or food processor. Add pecans, spoon into tart shells. Bake at 350 degrees for 25 minutes.

Yield . . . .   24 tarts

Calories for crust 52
Protein 1
Carbs. 4
Fat 3

Calories for filling 152
Protein 2
Carbs. 19
Fat 7

Total calories for entire tart . .204
Protein 3
Carbs. 23
Fat 10

STRAWBERRY TARTS

¼ cup melted butter
½ cup softened butter
½ cup Sweet Cloud Rice Syrup
2 eggs
½ cup ground almonds
1½ tsp. grated lemon rind
1½ cups unbleached white flour
1½ cups whole wheat pastry flour
¼ tsp. salt
1 tsp. vanilla
1 jar Westbrae Natural Strawberry Conserves (9 oz.)
1 cup fresh strawberries

Cream ½ cup softened butter and rice syrup. Beat in eggs, one at a time. Add almonds, lemon rind, and vanilla. Mix well. Add flour and salt slowly, mixing in well. Batter will be thick. Form into large ball. Cover and refrigerate for 1 hour.

Divide dough into 7 equal parts. Grease detached bottom of 10" spring form pan. Roll dough 1 part at a time; dough should be very thin. Cut to fit spring form pan, place one layer of dough on bottom section of pan.

Brush with butter, and spread 1 Tbsp. of jam over layer. Repeat until all dough is used. Top with remaining jam. Place ring around pan, place on cookie sheet. Bake at 400 degrees for 40-45 minutes, cool 5 minutes. Remove ring from pan, cool completely.

Ice with 8 Minute Frosting. Garnish with fresh strawberries over top.

Yield .... 27 — 1"pieces
Calories 184
Protein 3
Carbs. 29
Fat 7

STRAWBERRY LIGHT CREPES

¾ cup nonfat milk
1 egg
1 Tbsp. olive oil
⅛ tsp. ground nutmeg
½ cup whole wheat pastry flour
½ tsp. vanilla

In a small bowl combine all ingredients except flour. Mix well. Slowly add flour, mixing well after each addition. Over a hot grill sprayed with Pam, pour 2 Tbsp. batter making crepes as thin as possible.

Cook until the edges and bottom are golden brown, about 1 minute, flip over and continue to cook about 30 seconds. Do not overcook. Fill with strawberry filling (see next recipe), top with whipped cream.

STRAWBERRY FILLING

1 cup fresh strawberries (washed & drained)
1 cup whipping cream, whipped until stiff
¼ cup Sweet Cloud Rice Syrup

Pour rice syrup over strawberries, mix in whip cream. Fill crepes and fold in half, top with whipped cream.

```
Yield  ..............  10 crepes
Calories  .........134
Protein  ...........4
Carbs.  ...........10
Fat  ..............10
```

STRAWBERRY SHORT-COOKIE

3 Oat Bran Muffin Frookie's Cookies (By R. W. Frookie)
½ cup fresh strawberries
2 Tbsp. nonfat yogurt

Crumble cookies in serving dish. Spoon sliced strawberries over cookies. Top with yogurt.

```
Yield  .............   Serves 1
Calories  ........187
Protein  ...........2
Carbs.  ..........30
Fat  ..............6
```

CRISPY CAROB CHIP COOKIES

2 sticks (1 cup) softened butter
1 jar chilled Sweet Cloud Rice Syrup
1 Tbsp. vanilla
2 large eggs
2½ cups whole wheat pastry flour
1 tsp. salt
2 tsp. baking powder
2 Tbsp. ground coriander
4 cups walnut pieces
3 cups unsweetened carob chips

In mixing bowl, cream butter and rice syrup. Add vanilla. Mix well. Add eggs one at a time, mixing well with each addition.

Combine flour, salt, baking powder, and coriander. Slowly add this to butter & egg mixture, mixing well. Fold in walnuts and carob chips. Chill mixture for 1 hour. Drop cookies onto cookie sheet sprayed with Pam. Preheat oven to 375 degrees, bake 12 to 15 minutes.

Yield . . . .   9 dozen cookies
Calories 77
Protein 2
Carbs. 7
Fat 5

OATMEAL COOKIES

2 beaten eggs
1 cup uncooked old fashioned oatmeal
½ cup softened butter
¼ cup whole wheat flour
1 cup wheat germ
2 Tbsp. vanilla extract
¼ cup low-fat buttermilk
1 Tbsp. cinnamon
3 Tbsp. rice syrup
1 cup chopped pecans

Combine all ingredients, mix well. Roll batter into small balls. Bake at 350 degrees for 12 to 15 minutes.

Yield .... 4 dozen cookies
Calories 67
Protein 2
Carbs. 6
Fat 5

DATE BARS

¼ cup softened butter
2 eggs
1 tsp. grated orange rind
2 tsp. vanilla
1 cup whole wheat flour
2 tsp. baking powder
¼ tsp. salt
1 cup chopped dates (approx. 10 dates)
½ cup chopped walnuts

Cream butter and eggs, add orange rind and vanilla. Mix well. Add dates, mix well. Mix together flour, baking powder and salt. Add to egg mixture. Fold in nuts. Pour into a 9" X 9" X 2" square pan that has been sprayed with Pam. Bake at 350 degrees for 30 minutes or until golden brown. Chill and cut into bars.

Yield 16
Calories 99
Protein 2
Carbs. 10
Fat 6

DATE APPLE CRISP

3 medium unpeeled and sliced apples (approx. 1 lb.)
½ cup whole wheat flour
½ cup uncooked oatmeal
1 tsp. cinnamon
1 tsp. ground nutmeg
¼ tsp. salt (optional)
1 cup dates (approx. 10)
½ cup low-fat buttermilk
½ cup chopped pecans
¼ cup water

Preheat oven to 375 degrees. Use a 9" X 13" square pan sprayed with Pam and place in oven until hot. Remove from oven, arrange sliced apples in a row, set aside.

Mix dry ingredients and nuts together, set aside. Blend water, dates, and milk. Mix well. Mix date mixture with flour. Spread over apples being careful not to displace the apples. Bake at 375 degrees for 35 to 40 minutes or until golden brown.

```
Yield  . . . . . . . . . . . . .   12 squares
Calories  . . . . . . . . . .89
Protein . . . . . . . . . . .3
Carbs.   . . . . . . . . . .19
Fat   . . . . . . . . . . . . . .1
```

COCONUT CLUSTERS

1 cup fresh lightly toasted grated coconut
6 tsp. Premium Protein Powder (Neo-Life product)
1 cup chopped pecans
1 cup water
1 cup unsweetened carob chips
1 cup dates
½ cup nonfat milk
1 Tbsp. melted butter
1 tsp. vanilla

In blender or food processor, process dates, butter and milk well, set aside. In a heavy pot bring water to boil, lower heat and add carob chips. Stir constantly until creamy. Remove from heat, add vanilla and date mixture. Mix well. Let cool.

In a bowl, mix coconut, Protein Powder, and pecans. Pour carob-date mixture over coconut. Spoon out in clusters over wax paper on cookie sheet. Place in refrigerator to chill about 2 hours.

Yield . . . . 24 clusters
Calories 113
Protein 3
Carbs. 9
Fat 8

PECAN PRALINES

1 cup lowfat milk
1 — 15 oz. jar Sweet Cloud Rice Syrup
1 tsp. vanilla
1 Tbsp. softened butter
2 cups lightly roasted pecan halves

In a 4 quart saucepan, combine milk and rice syrup. Mix well over medium heat until milk and syrup comes to a boil. Cook to soft boil stage, about 234 degrees (mixture forms a ball when dropped into a cup of cold water). Remove from heat. Add vanilla and butter, mixing well. Continue to stir until mixture becomes slightly thickened. Add pecans and beat until mixture loses its gloss. Do not overbeat. Drop by heaping tablespoons on buttered platter. (If mixture becomes too thick, add a few drops of hot water.) Cool.

Yield .... 12 pralines
Calories 324
Protein 3
Carbs. 48
Fat 15

PEANUT BUTTER CAROB FUDGE

½ cup fruit sweetener
½ cup milk or Edensoy milk substitute
1 cup unsweetened carob chips
2 Tbsp. peanut butter (no sugar kind)
1 tsp. vanilla
1 Tbsp. softened butter
1 cup chopped pecans

Bring fruit sweetener and milk to boil. Add carob chips and peanut butter. Stir constantly until smooth. Remove from heat. Add vanilla and butter, mix well until slightly cooled. Fold in pecans, then place in 9" buttered square pan. Refrigerate for about 1 hour or until set. Cut into squares.

```
Yield  . . . . . . . . . . . . . .   24 squares
Calories  . . . . . . . . . .87
Protein  . . . . . . . . . . . .3
Carbs.   . . . . . . . . . . . .8
Fat   . . . . . . . . . . . . . .6
```

DIVINITY

1 — 15 oz. jar Sweet Cloud Rice Syrup
½ cup water
¼ tsp. salt
3 egg whites
¼ tsp. cream of tartar
1 tsp. vanilla
1 cup lightly toasted chopped pecans

Mix together rice syrup, water, and salt in a 2 quart glass bowl. Cook in microwave on high for 18-20 minutes, stirring every 5 minutes. (Mixture should appear thick but not candied.) During the last three minutes, while syrup is cooking, beat egg whites with cream of tartar until very stiff.

Gradually pour hot syrup over egg whites, continue beating at high speed until mixture thickens and starts to lose its gloss, about 12-15 minutes. Add vanilla. Mix well. Fold in nuts and drop by teaspoonful onto wax paper. Refrigerate approximately 2 hours or until firm.

Yield .... 2 dozen
Calories 122
Protein 1
Carbs. 23
Fat 4

CHOCOLATE ECLAIRS

POPOVERS

1 cup whole wheat flour
¼ tsp. salt
3 eggs
1 Tbsp. melted butter
1 cup low-fat buttermilk
2 Tbsp. butter, cut into 6 small pieces

Spray popover pan with Pam. Preheat oven to 425 degrees. Set rack in middle of oven for about 2 minutes. Blend ingredients together at high speed in mixer or food processor for about 4 minutes. Batter should be very smooth.

Place small pieces of butter in popover pan to melt (return to oven about 1 minute to melt butter). Fill each cup ½ full with batter and bake at 400 degrees for 20 minutes, then lower heat to 350 degrees for 30-40 minutes, or until popover tests done. Remove from oven. Set aside to cool. (See next recipe for filling.)

Filling

2 cups nonfat milk
2 egg yolks
1 Tbsp. whole wheat flour
1 tsp. vanilla
1 tsp. chocolate extract
¼ cup carob powder
½ cup Sweet Cloud Rice Syrup

In heavy pot cook milk, egg yolks, flour, and carob powder over medium heat until thick. Remove from heat. Add vanilla, chocolate extract, and rice syrup, mixing well. Set in refrigerator about 15 minutes to cool. Mixture should be slightly thickened, but not too thick.

Fill basting bulb with filling and insert into side of popover and squeeze. Fill each popover and return to refrigerator for about 3 hours before serving.

Yield . . . . Serves 6
Calories — Popovers only . . .187
Protein 7
Carbs. 17
Fat 10

Calories — Filling only . . .77
Protein 4
Carbs. 9
Fat 3

Total Eclair Calories 264
Protein .11
Carbs. 26
Fat 13

WHIP CREAM TOPPING

½ pint whipping cream
1 tsp. vanilla
2 Tbsp. Sweet Cloud Rice Syrup

    Combine ingredients. Whip at high speed with a mixer until thick. Chill.

Yield	Approx. 12 Tbsp. — 1 cup
Serving Size	1 Tbsp.
Calories 58	
Protein 4	
Carbs. ....trace	
Fat 6	

STRAWBERRY YOGURT ICE CREAM

1 cup evaporated skim milk
3 cups nonfat yogurt
2 cups nonfat powdered milk
    (powdered form — DO NOT MIX WITH WATER)
1 pkg. Sugar-Free Strawberry Jello
2 Tbsp. vanilla flavoring
2 cups frozen fresh strawberries (no sugar kind)

Blend all ingredients except strawberries in blender until smooth. Add strawberries, blend slightly. Place in electric Ice Cream Freezer to make.

Yield .... 10 cups
Serving Size .... ½ cup
Calories 76
Protein 6
Carbs. 13
Fat ..less than 1 gram

COOKIES AND CREAM

2 dozen Carob Chip Cookies
approx. 1 gallon Vanilla Ice Cream — See Recipe
2 cups Whip Cream Topping — See Recipe
½ cup lightly roasted chopped pecans
½ cup lightly roasted chopped walnuts

In a 9" X 13" baking dish, crumble carob chip cookies evenly, top with Vanilla ice cream. Cover with foil, place in freezer for 2 hours. Mix whipping cream until stiff. Spread over ice cream evenly. Cover and return to freezer for approximately 4 hours. Top with roasted nuts before serving.

```
Yield  .............. 12 — 1½" X 2" pieces
Calories .........464
Protein ............. 14
Carbs.  ............. 39
Fat  ............... 39
```

VANILLA ICE CREAM

1 cup heavy whipping cream
3 cans evaporated skim milk
3 eggs
1⅓ cup instant nonfat dry milk
    (Powder form — DO NOT MIX WITH WATER)
1 Tbsp. vanilla
1 pkg. Sugar-free instant vanilla pudding mix
1 cup Sweet Cloud Rice Syrup

In blender, mix all ingredients. (Fresh fruit may be added if desired). Make in ice cream freezer.

Yield .... approx. 1 gallon
Serving Size .... ¼ cup = 1 scoop
Calories 182
Protein 7
Carbs. 16
Fat 10

EASY FROZEN YOGURT

1 frozen banana (wrap in Saran wrap then place in freezer)
½ cup plain nonfat yogurt (no sugar kind)
¼ cup unsweetened pineapple juice
½ cup fresh or frozen strawberries (no sugar)
1 tsp. vanilla
2 Tsp. Sweet Cloud Rice Syrup

Slice banana, place all ingredients in blender on high. Spoon into individual serving dishes. Freeze until firm, about 30 minutes. Serve with chopped nuts over the top. A little fresh fruit may also be added.

Yield .... Serves 4
Calories 57
Protein 2
Carbs. 22
Fat 0

BANANA SPLIT

½ medium banana, cut in half
3 scoops homemade Vanilla Ice Cream (See recipe)
2 Tbsp. crushed unsweetened pineapple
2 Tbsp. fresh mashed strawberries
1 Tbsp. carob topping (See recipe)
1 Tbsp. chopped pecans
2 fresh chopped cherries

Place halved banana in ice cream dish. Arrange Vanilla Ice Cream scoops in center of banana, then top with Carob Topping and fruit. Sprinkle with nuts and cherries. (Top with Whip Cream Topping if desired.)

```
Yield ..............   Serves 1
Calories  ........ 782
Protein  .......... 24
Carbs. ........... 82
Fat .............. 42
```

CAROB FUDGE ICE CREAM SUNDAE

½ cup homemade Vanilla Ice Cream (See recipe)
2 Tbsp. Carob Topping (See recipe)
1 Tbsp. chopped pecans
2 fresh chopped cherries

Place Vanilla Ice Cream in dish, top with Carob Topping, nuts, and cherries.

Yield . . . .   Serves 1
Calories 629
Protein 19
Carbs. 59
Fat 37

CAROB TOPPING

½ cup water
1 cup unsweetened carob chips
1 tsp. butter
1 tsp. vanilla
¼ cup Sweet Cloud Rice Syrup

Bring water to boil. Add carob chips, stirring constantly until smooth and creamy. Remove from fire. Stir in butter, vanilla, and rice syrup. Can be stored in refrigerator and reheated before using.

Yield	1 cup
Serving Size	1 Tbsp.
Calories 96	
Protein 2	
Carbs. 11	
Fat 5	

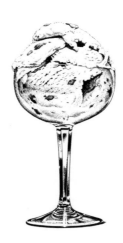

Miscellaneous

PARTY PUNCH

Juice of 1 lemon
Juice of 4 oranges
4 cups unsweetened pineapple juice
1 jar cranberry juice (from health food store)
1 bottle sparkling apple cider
2 cups water
1 cup fresh strawberries (optional)

Mix all ingredients together in punch bowl. Fresh strawberries may be added to float in punch.

Serving Size .... 1 cup
Calories 87
Protein 1
Carbs. 22
Fat 0

ICED HERB TEA

2 cups herb tea (any kind)
juice of 1 orange
juice of 1 lemon
1 Tbsp. Fruit Sweetener

Mix together and serve over ice.

Calories 85
Protein 2
Carbs. 22
Fat 0

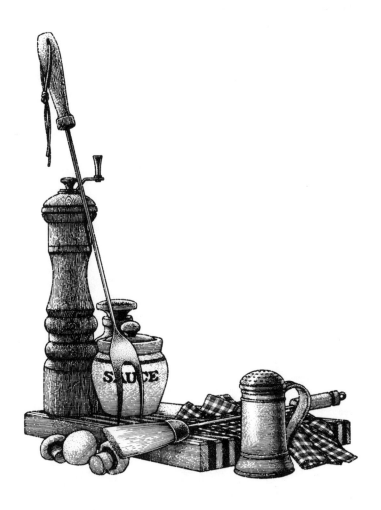

HOT CAROB COCOA

2 Tbsp. carob powder
¼ cup water
1 cup nonfat milk
¼ tsp. vanilla
1 Tbsp. Sweet Cloud Rice Syrup

Bring water, rice syrup and carob powder to boil. Add milk and mix well. Stir until heated. Remove from fire, stir in vanilla.

Calories 121
Protein 8
Carbs. 19
Fat 0

HOMEMADE MAPLE SYRUP

½ cup water
½ cup butter
1 pkg. Knox unflavored gelatin
½ tsp. vanilla flavoring (no sugar kind)
½ tsp. maple flavoring (no sugar kind)
¼ cup Fruit Sweetener

Bring water, fruit sweetener, and butter to a boil. Add gelatin and, stir until dissolved. Take off fire, add flavorings, stir well. Let cool a few minutes until slightly thick.

```
Yield  .............  1 cup
Serving Size  ........  1 Tbsp.
Calories  ..........68
Protein ............0
Carbs.  ............0
Fat  ..............8
```

STRAWBERRY SYRUP

½ cup water
½ cup butter
1 pkg. Knox unflavored gelatin
1 tsp. vanilla
2 Tbsp. Westbrae Natural Strawberry Conserves

Bring water, butter, and gelatin to boil. Add strawberry conserves, stirring constantly until dissolved. Remove from fire, add vanilla. Cool slightly before serving.

Yield .... 1 cup
Calories 73
Protein 0
Carbs. 2
Fat 8

REAL SYRUP

½ cup butter
1 tsp. vanilla
1 tsp. maple extract (no sugar)
1 — 15 oz. jar Sweet Cloud Rice Syrup

Melt butter in heavy pot. Stir in rice syrup. Remove from heat. Add vanilla and maple flavorings, mixing well. Serve over pancakes or French toast. Store in refrigerator.

Yield . . . . 1½ cups
Calories 103
Protein 0
Carbs. 15
Fat 8

STRAWBERRY JAM

¼ cup orange juice
1 cup mashed strawberries
1 pkg. Sugar Free Strawberry Jello
1 Tbsp. orange rind

Sprinkle gelatin over orange juice, let stand 5 minutes, then bring to a boil. Remove from fire. Pour over mashed strawberries. Mix well. Store in glass jar in refrigerator.

Serving Size . . . . 1 Tbsp.
Calories 7
Protein 0
Carbs. 2
Fat 0

CRANBERRY SAUCE

1 bag fresh cranberries
½ cup water
2 cups fruit sweetener
1 pkg. Knox unflavored gelatin

Bring cranberries, water, and sweeteners to a boil. Lower heat and simmer for 10 to 15 minutes. Dissolve gelatin into mixture. Remove from fire. Cranberries may be served whole or strained through a fine strainer. Chill before serving.

Serving Size .... 1 Tbsp.
Calories 46
Protein 0
Carbs. 11
Fat 0

HOMEMADE BARBECUE SAUCE

3 lbs. onions
1 cup celery
2 large bell peppers
½ cup Bread & Butter Pickles (homemade or use no sugar dill pickles)
1 — 10 ⅘ oz. can tomato puree
2 cups olive oil
1 Tbsp. prepared mustard
1 — 3 oz. bottle Louisiana Hot Sauce
1 cup pimentos
4 cups water
1 cup fruit sweetener

Process onions, celery, bell peppers, and pickles in food processor or blender. Add to water and cook covered on low heat for 2 hours. Add remaining ingredients. Cook 1 more hour.

Place in sterile pint jars or Ziploc bags for freezing.

```
Yield  . . . . . . . . . . . . . .   4 quarts
Serving Size  . . . . . . . .   1 Tbsp.
Calories  . . . . . . . . . .41
Protein . . . . . . . . . . . .0
Carbs.  . . . . . . . . . . . .3
Fat  . . . . . . . . . . . . . .4
```

ITALIAN BREAD CRUMBS

2 cups Nutri-Grain wheat cereal
½ tsp. garlic powder
1 tsp. Italian herb seasoning
1 tsp. oregano leaves
½ tsp. pepper
¼ tsp. salt

Blend cereal in blender until powdered. Add seasonings, mix well. If toasted crumbs are needed, add 3 Tbsp. butter and bake in oven for 10 minutes or until brown.

Yield .... Approx. 16 Tbsp.
Serving Size .... 1 Tbsp.
Calories 16
Protein 5
Carbs. 4
Fat 0

BREAD AND BUTTER PICKLES

4 cups sliced cucumbers (about 8 cucumbers)
1 cup sliced onions
1¼ cups cider vinegar
½ tsp. tumeric
½ tsp. mustard seed
¼ tsp. celery seed
¼ cup Fruit Sweetener

Combine cucumbers and onions. Cover with ice and let stand for 3 hours, then drain. Combine vinegar, spices, and fruit sweetener, bring to a boil. Add cucumber mixture and heat about 3 minutes. Remove from heat. Stir until dissolved. Serve chilled. Pickles may be canned and stored.

PESTO PASTA SAUCE DRESSING

1 pkg. Mayacamas Brand Pesto Pasta Sauce Mix
4 oz. hot water
1 Tbsp. olive oil
1 Tbsp. parmesan cheese

Mix all ingredients in pint jar. Mix well. Store in refrigerator.

Yield .... 1 cup
Serving Size .... 1 Tbsp.
Calories 12
Protein ....trace
Carbs. ....trace
Fat 1

HOT CAROB DRINK

8 oz. Westsoy Lite — plain Natural soy drink
3 Tbsp. carob powder
½ tsp. vanilla
1 Tbsp. fruit sweetener

Heat soy drink in pot. Mix carob powder in well. When heated through, add vanilla and fruit sweetener. Mix well. Serve hot.

Calories 253
Protein 5
Carbs. 53
Fat 2

BANANA SOY SLUSH

8 oz. Westsoy Lite-plain Natural soy drink
½ frozen banana
ice cubes

Mix all ingredients in blender until smooth.

Calories 153
Protein 5
Carbs.   30
Fat   2

BERRY SAUCE

2 cups fresh strawberries (blueberries may be substituted)
1 Tbsp. lemon juice
¼ tsp. lemon rind
2 tsp. whole wheat flour
2 Tbsp. water

Cook berries until very hot. Add lemon juice, & grated lemon rind. Simmer 5 minutes. Force through a sieve.

Mix together flour and water until smooth. Add berry mixture and cook over low heat, stirring constantly until it is clear and thickened.

Sauce may be served hot or cold.

Serve over fruit or ice cream.

Yield .... 1½ cups
Calories 119
Protein 3
Carbs. 24
Fat 0

CHAPTER 11

STAYING ON THE PROGRAM

Attitudes

Some people tell me it is too much trouble to read all the product labels or to be so careful when you go out to eat. To this I say, "You don't feel bad enough." That is why it is too much trouble. Human nature is funny. If we still have a few good days, we can put up with the bad days and accept them. Most of us have to reach a point in our lives where we can't go on anymore. We feel as if we will die if something doesn't change. Only when we realize that there aren't any good days anymore, do we do something about our condition and realize that major changes have to be made. That was the point I had reached when I decided that there had to be a better way of life. I just couldn't go on living that way. We are all creatures of habit, and it isn't easy to change.

Some people tell me they can't afford it. The better-quality food costs too much or the vitamins are too expensive. The way I look at it, you can't afford not to take a healthier approach. Consider what you are spending now on doctor bills, or hospital bills, and on the drugs you are taking. Consider the results you are getting. With all that you are spending, is it making you feel better? I doubt it, or you wouldn't be reading this book.

What I offer you isn't easy, but you get results and you can't put a price tag on good health.

Family Cooperation

Some people blame their spouses or family members because they can't stay with my program. The family won't accept eating the way you have to and it is too hard to fix two different meals. I agree that it is too much trouble to continue doing this for a long time. You will not be able to change your family's bad eating habits overnight. If you try, they may sabotage your kitchen and remove you as head cook. So use a little tact. For instance, when you cook rice, cook one pot of white rice and one pot of brown rice. Then mix them together. You will eat only the brown rice, but give your family the mixture. As they get used to the texture of the brown rice, cut back on the amount of the white rice and in time they will not complain when you serve only the brown rice. In fact, they will love it! It takes a while to get used to the texture. As a Louisiana Cajun, I love my rice and gravy. At first I had to make myself eat the brown rice. I would tell myself, "it's good for you, so eat it." After a while, I realized I was enjoying rice much more than ever before. I tried eating a little white rice and realized how gummy it was. It would stick to the roof of my mouth. I was amazed that I had never noticed this before.

The same goes for pancakes, use unbleached white flour, mixed with a little whole wheat flour, and again as your family gets accustomed to the texture, add more whole wheat flour. Before long they will not realize they are eating healthy foods. Continue to bake them desserts like you used to, but now and then substitute one of the desserts in this book. You don't have to tell them it doesn't have sugar in it. If you do, they will immediately decide they don't like it. Pretend it is a new recipe you thought they might like.

In time, you will be surprised with the results. Use a little tact. Be a little sneaky; they will thank you for it later and never know what hit them. Sometimes the family we love so much and want to help the most are the ones who will give us the most trouble when we try to introduce changes.

Success Means Forever

The pay-off for being successful in my program is that I have gotten my life back. I lived too many years in a fog, with restrictions and limitations. I can no longer accept that way of living.

With my busy schedule I cannot afford to let poor health get in my way. As a professional fitness trainer and a therapist, I have too many people depending on my ability to help them with their needs to worry about my mood swings or headaches.

Much has happened in my life since those early years of confusion and temptation. I no longer feel as though I have to focus my entire concentration on myself. Without realizing what was happening, all the pieces have come together like a well-worked puzzle on a rainy day. The program is that easy for me now, but it was a long time getting there.

After many years of counseling diabetics and hypoglycemics, I can easily understand the confusion they feel when confronted with having to make major changes in their life styles in order to achieve a healthier more productive life. I see the doubt in their eyes when I tell them it will get easier in time.

Often it is simply a matter of removing temptation from our paths. One diabetic client working in a bakery found she was completely powerless when it came to avoiding the leftover icing at the end of the day. I too could remember when the icing was my favorite part of a birthday cake from Joe's Party House. As sure as I am of myself, I don't know if I could trust myself were I in her position. The obvious choice for that diabetic client was to find another job, farther away from her temptation.

I am sometimes amused with the interpretation clients somtimes have on my recommendations. One lady, when told she could choose to have the fruit-juice-sweetened candy bars instead of the one containing sugar, decided half of one wasn't enough, she ended up eating five at one time. On her follow-up visit she informed me she couldn't understand why she had such a problem with the candy when I had told her she should have been able to tolerate it. From then on, I made myself clear when discussing portion control with fruit-juice-sweetened products. Even with allowed foods, it is important to use common sense with the portions one is able to tolerate.

From time to time a client will stray off the program, but most will return. With time they realize nothing else will work as well. One client returned after eight years, reporting he could no longer tolerate the mood swings and mental confusion. After going through a divorce, he realized he had to put himself back on track if he was ever going to live a normal life again. After all these years it wasn't easy to take the necessary steps needed to control his blood sugar, especially since he no longer had a spouse to help him with the meal planning.

Sometimes we no longer have a choice—we have to do it. Somehow we believe we are exempt from the problems that go along with poor nutritional habits. All too often this kind of behavior catches up with us.

But we are, after all, only human, and we can only keep trying until we get it right.

Start the program and stay on it. If you have a lapse, don't get mired in guilt; forgive yourself, and get back on track.

I know you can do it. All you need is to start to grow a "seed of confidence" within yourself. What I mean by this is that as soon as you see the first changes, the first improvements in how you feel, you will begin to feel a little bit confident about the program and your ability to stick with it. You will begin to believe that you really can change your life.

This "seed of confidence" will grow with each improvement you make. As you continue, you will gradually begin to master the skills of nutritious, healthy eating, fitness and weight control until, finally, nothing can shake your belief in yourself—that the rest of your life is going to be healthy, energetic and fruitful.

Welcome to the program! Welcome to life!

APPENDIX A

Hypoglycemia Questionnaire

Signs & Symptoms of Hypoglycemia

Check each symptom according to its severity, as follows.
The problem:
  Column 1 - never occurs (mark o)
  Column 2 - is mild and occurs occasionally (check if applies)
  Column 3 - is moderate and/or occurs at least once a week (check if applies)
  Column 4 - is severe and occurs frequently (check if applies)

Column No.

1	2	3	4	
				Can't concentrate
				Can't make decisions
				Can't get started in the morning
				Can't work well under pressure
				Consume excessive alcohol
				Crave candy, soda, or coffee between meals or mid afternoon
				Cry easily, or feel like crying inside
				Depressed
				Drink more than three cups of coffee or cola drinks daily
				Eat candy, cake or drink soda pop
				Eat bread, pasta, potatoes, rice, or beans
				Eat when nervous
				Eat without feeling hunger
				Fearful (Overwhelmed by people, places or things)
				Feel insecure or have a low self-image

Column No.

1	2	3	4	
				Fits or anger
				Headaches
				Highly emotional
				Hungry between meals or at night
				Insomnia, awakening with inability to return to sleep
				Lack of energy
				Magnify insignificant details
				Moody
				Poor memory
				Reduced initiative
				Sleepy during the day
				Sleepy or drowsy after meals
				Tired most of the time
				Wake up after a few hours sleep
				Worry frequently
				Allergies: asthma, hay fever, skin rash, sinus trouble, etc.
				Bad dreams
				Bleeding gums
				Blurred vision
				Bored
				Bruise easily
				Cold hands or feet (even during summertime)
				Convulsions
				Dizziness, giddiness, or light-headedness
				Fatigue relieved by eating
				Feel faint if meal is delayed
				Get shaky inside when hungry
				Hallucinations
				Having the need to sigh
				Heart beats fast (palpitations)

Column No.

1	2	3	4	
				Irritable before meals
				Muscle twitching or cramps
				Phobias (excessive fear of something or situation)
				Reduced sex drive
				Skin aches or itches
				Stomach cramps or "nervous stomach"
				Suicidal thoughts or tendencies: feeling of hopelessness
				Sweating excessively
				Trembling (shaking) of the hands
				Ulcers, gastritis, chronic indigestion, abdominal bloating
				Uncoordinated (drop or bump into things)
				Unsocial or antisocial behavior
				Total number of checks in each column

Multiply total checks in each column by Column No.

_____ X 1 = _____   _____ X 2 = _____

_____ X 3 = _____   _____ X 4 = _____

GRAND TOTAL: _____

(For example: If you have 15 checks in Column No. 3. Multiply 15 times 3. Do the same for each column)

GRAND TOTAL OF:

0 - 15	5% PROBABILITY OF HAVING HYPOGLYCEMIA
16 - 20	15% PROBABILITY OF HAVING HYPOGLYCEMIA
21 - 25	50% PROBABILITY OF HAVING HYPOGLYCEMIA
26 - 35	75% PROBABILITY OF HAVING HYPOGLYCEMIA
36 - 45	90% PROBABILITY OF HAVING HYPOGLYCEMIA
46+	98% PROBABILITY OF HAVING HYPOGLYCEMIA

Diabetes Questionnaire

Signs & Syptoms of Diabetes

Points

1. 10 - Blood glucose Above 140 mg/dl
2. 4 - Unquenchable thirst (more than 10 glasses per day)
3. 4 - Frequent urination expecially during the night
4. 2 - Wounds that will not heal
5. 3 - Numbness and tingling of the feet
6. 2 - Hands and feet are itching
7. 2 - Feeling of severe fatigue
8. 2 - Always hungry (especially after eating)
9. 2 - Unexplained weight gain or weight loss
10. 2 - Overweight or overfat
11. 2 - Sexual dysfunctions
12. 3 - Vaginal infections (itching/yeast infections)
13. 2 - Family history of diabetes

ADD THE TOTAL POINTS OF SYMPTOMS THAT APPLY TO YOU.

IF YOUR TOTAL EQUALS 7 OR MORE,

THIS IS A POSSIBLE INDICATION OF DIABETES.

IF SO, SEE YOUR DOCTOR.

APPENDIX B

Vitamins and Other Supplements

Beta Carotene:
(A form of Vitamin A)— 25,000 IU per day

* A fat soluble vitamin

Benefits:

1. Counteract night blindness, weak eyesight, and can be helpful in the treatment of eye disorders.
2. Protects mucous membranes, reducing susceptibility to infection and builds resistance to respiratory disease.
3. Protects soft tissues.
4. Promotes secretion of gastric juices.
5. Builds strong bones and teeth.
6. Helps in the removal of age spots.
7. Helps in the treatment of acne, impetigo, boils, carbuncles, and open ulcers. Can also be applied externally for additional benefits.

- *Good food sources:* Fish, fish liver oils, carrots, green and yellow vegetables, yellow fruits, and sweet potatoes.
- *Works best in conjunction with:* Zinc, B-Complex, Vitamin D, Vitamin E, Calcium, and Phosphorus.

Vitamin B-Complex:

50 mg.- Balanced formula- once daily

* A water soluble vitamin

Benefits:

1. Helps maintain a healthy nervous system.

2. An aid in managing stress.

3. Stabilizes appetite by improving digestion.

4. Necessary for the production of stomach acid.

5. Needed for the breakdown of carbohydrates, fats, and proteins.

6. Maintains healthy skin, nails and hair.

7. Helps in reducing cholesterol levels in blood.

8. Assists in the production and utilization of fatty acids.

9. Helps preserve stored Vitamin A.

10. Helps in eliminating sore mouths, lips, and tongue. Prevents edge of mouth from cracking.

- *Good food sources:* Brewer's yeast, whole grains, brown rice, fish, legumes, nuts, seeds, wheat germ, green leafy vegetables, and root vegetables.

- **Works best when taken in a balanced form.** If other B vitamins are taken, always take a B-Complex with it to prevent deficiencies. Take Iron with it to better insure proper metabolization.

Other B Vitamins:

B-6: 250 mg. per day.
B-12: 1-3 cc., one to three times per week.
Folic Acid: 400 mcg., 1 mg. per day.
Pantothenic Acid, 200-500 mg. per day.

Vitamin C:

500-3000 mg. per day, or up to bowel tolerance

* A water soluble vitamin.

Benefits:

1. Maintains collagen, a protein necessary in skin, bone, ligaments, and other tissues.

2. Helps in body's absorption of iron.

3. Helps fight infection.

4. Protects against oxidation.

5. Helps in managing stress.

6. Reduces allergy reactions.

7. Strengthens capillaries and connective tissue and helpful in preventing hemorrhage.

8. Helps in decreasing blood cholesterol.

9. Helps counteract the formation of nitrosamine (a cancer causing substance found in meats and other foods.)

10. Aids in treatment and prevention of common colds.

- *Good food sources:* Citrus fruit, rose hips, acerola cherries, sprouted alfalfa seeds, cantaloupe, strawberries, green and leafy vegetables, broccoli, and green peppers.

- **Works best in conjunction with:** Calcium and magnesium, taken with bioflavonoids. Large doses of Ascorbic Acid can upset the gastrointestinal tract. For this reason, it is recommended that you use only Vitamin C from a natural food source. In the natural formulation, you will receive the C complex of bioflavonoids, hesperidin, and rutin. Diabetics need to be aware that when testing the urine for sugar, it could be inaccurate if you are taking large amounts of Vitamin C. Ask your physician or pharmacist for the proper testing kit not affected by Vitamin C.

Vitamin E:
400-800 IU per day

  * An oil soluble vitamin

Benefits:

1. An antioxidant, plays a vital role in free radical pathology.

2. Markedly increases the endurance during heavy exercise.

3. Essential to cellular respiration in muscles.

4. Aids in dilation of blood vessels.

5. Prevents clot formation.

6. Helps prevent scar formation.

7. Keeps one looking younger by retarding cellular aging through oxidation.

8. Helps accelerate healing of burns.

9. Helps alleviate leg cramps when taken along with calcium.

10. Helpful in regulating hormones.

- **Works best when taken in conjunction with:** Selenium. Also works well with Vitamin A to protect lungs against air pollution. It is composed of compounds called tocopherols, Alpha, beta, gamma, delta, epsilon, zeta, eta, and theta. Most effective when taken in a 100% natural base which includes all eight tocopherols. Vitamin E is best not taken with inorganic iron (ferrous sulfate).

  If an iron supplement is recommended, use only an organic iron complex such as Ferrous gluconate, peptonate, citrate, or fumarate. These do not destroy Vitamin E.

- **Good food sources:** Wheat germ, soybeans, vegetable oils, broccoli, brussels sprouts, leafy greens, spinach, whole wheat flour, whole-grain cereals, and raw nuts.

Iron:
25mg. per day

* A mineral.

Benefits:

1. Necessary for normal energy flow at the cellular level.

2. Helps protein metabolism.

3. Needed for formation of hemoglobin.

4. Improves respiratory action.

5. Prevents fatigue.

6. Aids in promoting resistance to disease.

- *Works best in conjunction with:* Vitamin C, copper, cobalt, manganese, necessary for proper assimilation. Use an organic iron such as ferrous gluconate, ferrous fumarate, ferrous citrate, or ferrous peptonate, in a chelated form.

- *Good food sources:* Dried peaches, nuts, beans, asparagus, black strap molasses, oatmeal, and dark green vegetables, such as spinach.

Magnesium:
400-800 mg. per day

* A mineral.

Benefits:

1. Works with calcium as a natural tranquilizer.
2. Helps to promote a healthier cardiovascular system and helps prevent heart attacks.
3. Protects against kidney stones and gallstones by preventing calcium deposits from forming.
4. Helps convert blood sugar into energy.
5. Necessary for Vitamin C and Calcium metabolism.
6. Essential for effective nerve and muscle functions.
7. Considered the anti-stress mineral.

- *Works best with:* Calcium, Vitamin A, and phosphorus.
- *Good food sources:* Whole-grain cereals, figs, lemons, grapefruit, yellow corn, almonds, nuts, seeds, dark green vegetables, apples, kelp, and seafood.

Selenium:
100 mcg per day

* A mineral

Benefits:

1. Works with Vitamin E to protect membranes from damage.

2. Promotes normal body growth.

3. Acts as an antioxidant, along with Vitamin E.

4. Helps protect the body against cancer.

5. Helps maintain tissue elasticity.

6. Helps alleviate hot flashes and menopausal distress.

7. Helps in the treatment and prevention of dandruff.

8. Helpful in slowing down the aging process.

- *Works best with:* Vitamin E.
- *Good food sources:* Wheat germ, bran, tuna fish, garlic, onions, tomatoes, and broccoli.

Zinc:
25-50 mg. three times per day.

* A mineral

Benefits:

1. Involved in over twenty-five enzyme systems.

2. Activates B-Complex and Vitamin A.

3. Aids in wound healing and tissue repair.

4. Essential for protein synthesis.

5. Helps in the formation of insulin.

6. Aids in muscle contractibility.

7. Aids in the health of the prostate and important in development of all reproductive organs.

8. Important in brain function and mental alertness.

9. Gets rid of white spots and lines on fingernails.

10. Helps improve the sense of taste and smell.

11. Helps in decreasing cholesterol deposits.

- *Works best with:* Vitamin A, calcium and phosphorus.

NOTE: Zinc, as with all minerals, is more easily absorbed when taken in the chelated form.

- *Good food sources:* Whole grains, brewer's yeast, pumpkin seeds, sunflower seeds, and ground mustard.

Chromium:
100-200 mcg. per day

* A mineral.

Benefits:

1. Works with insulin in the metabolization of sugar.
2. Helps distribute protein where it is needed.
3. Designated as the glucose tolerance factor.(GTF)
4. Helps in metabolization of glucose for energy.
5. Aids in lowering high blood pressure.
6. Works as a deterrent for diabetes and arteriosclerosis.
7. Helps transport glucose into cells.

- *Works best:* If taken with the glucose tolerance factor. (GTF)
- *Good food sources:* Corn oil, brewer's yeast, whole grain cereals.

Calcium:
Women-1800-2000 mg. per day,
Men-1000-1800 mg. per day.

* A mineral

Benefits:

1. Calcium and phosphorous work together for healthy bones and teeth.
2. Calcium and magnesium work together for cardiovascular fitness.
3. Helps maintain strong bones and teeth.

4. Helpful in alleviating insomnia, considered nature's tranquilizer.

5. Helpful in metabolizing the body's iron.

6. Aids in impulse transmission of the nervous system.

7. Prevents muscle cramps and spasms.

8. Helpful in relieving menstrual cramps.

9. Helpful with "growing pains," a problem some young children and teenagers have.

- *Works best with:* Vitamins A, C, D, iron, and magnesium

- *Good food sources:* Soybeans, sardines, salmon, walnuts, peanuts, almonds, sunflower seeds, all dried beans, and green vegetables.

- NOTE: Calcium is best taken between meals. A high fiber meal can interfere with its absorption. Part of your daily calcium should be taken at bedtime.

Lipids and Sterols:

These should be included in your multiple vitamins.

- **Digestive Aids:** Hydrochloric Acid (HCL)—1 to 3 tablets before meals.

- **Pancreatic Digestive Enzymes:** 1 to 3 tablets after meals.

- **Glandulars:** Raw Pituitary tablets.

- **Raw Adrenal tablets.**

- **Raw Thyroid, or Thyro-Stim.**

- **Kelp.**

In Summary:

WOMEN

Vitamin A -	2500 IU per day
Vitamin B Complex - (balanced formula)	2 - 3 per day
Vitamin C -	500 - 3000 mg per day (recc. bowel tolerance)
Vitamin E -	800 IU per day
Iron -	25 mg per day
Calcium/Magnesium -	1000 mg per day
	1500 mg for females over 50 years old
Multi Mineral Complex -	2 per day
Chromuim	100 mcg per day
Multi-Glandular Complex -	3 per day
Digestive Aids -	1 - 3 before meals
Digestive Enzymes -	1 - 3 after meals

MEN

Vitamin A -	25000 IU per day
Vitamin B Complex -	2 - 3 per day
Vitamin C -	500 - 3000 mg per day (up to bowel tolerance)
Vitamin E -	800 IU per day
Iron -	25 mg per day*
Calcium/Magnesium -	800 - 1000 mg per day
Multi-Mineral Complex -	2 - 3 per day
Chromuim -	100 mcg per day
Multi-Glandular Complex -	2 - 3 per day
Digestive Aids -	1 - 3 before meals
Digestive Enzymes -	1 - 3 after meals

*NOTE: For best absorption, all vitamins and minerals should be natural and organic.

The average person may find it more convenient to use a multi-vitamin preparation rather than to take each vitamin separately. We recommend the following brand names. These may be purchased through your local health food stores or through a Neo-Life distributor.

Brand Names:

Neo-Life "Stress 30" packets

Twin Labs "Duo Tabs"

Biotics "Multi-Glandula Formula"

For non-menstruation Females or Males: Solgar "Solovite"

Nature's Plus "Nutragenic"

* Please note that multi-vitamins are best taken with meals, and that they do not contain enough vitamin C.

APPENDIX C

SUPPORT GROUPS

HYPOGLYCEMIA

1. Hypoglycemic and Parents of Minors With Hypoglycemia
   Dr. John W. Tintera Memorial Hypoglycemia Lay Group
   149 Spindele Road
   Hicksville, NY 11801
   516-731-3302

2. National Hypoglycemia Association
   P.O. Box 120
   Ridgewood, NJ 07451
   201-670-1189
   Founder and Director - Lenore L. Cohen

DIABETES

1. American Diabetes Association
   National Center
   P.O. Box 25757
   1660 Duke St.
   Alexandra, VA 22314
   703-549-1500
   Director - Barbara Akin

Index

(OK To Photocopy This Order Form)

To order additional copies of:

Hypoglycemia and Diabetes Wellness Guide

by Freda Whalen, RMT and Gilbert Manso, M.D.

(ISBN 0-9638201-1-7)

Please fill out the form below.
Return it with payment for all orders. Thank you.

Send me _____ copies for a total cost of $_____.

Costs: $19.95 each, plus $4.50 for first book (S&H)
& $2.00 for each additional copy.
(Louisiana residents, add 8.5% sales tax.)

Save on large orders!

Order 5 copies for $79.95, plus shipping.
Order 10 copies for only $159.95, plus shipping.
For special pricing on large orders, contact publisher.

Ship Books To My Address Below:

Name: _____

Organization: _____

Address: _____

City: _____ State: _____ Zip: _____

Telephone: _____ Fax: _____

Order Books From The Publisher:

Body Care Publications
P. O. Box 5981 • Lake Charles, LA 70606
Telephone: 1-800-269-8460
FAX: (318) 497-0607

1